Waltzing With Jim Dancer

A Personal Tale of Survival.

Chapter one – Cancer… What cancer?

Being told you have cancer is a head fuck of the highest magnitude. While there are probably far more eloquent ways of describing the feeling that comes over the mind when one is told cancer is present in the body; for me… it was a head fuck, an 'Oh my God… I'm going to die!' feeling. There are no witty retorts, it is not possible to be nonchalant and there is nowhere to run to other than the big, blank wall that takes over your powers of thought. All I could do was sit there in stunned silence, waiting for the doctor to tell me he was only kidding, and to apologise for his sick sense of humour. I was far from ready to die. I was just coming up to my 51st birthday, barely middle-aged, and far too young to kick the bucket. I had read somewhere, probably on the Internet, that by the year 2050 people were going to be living as long as 150 years; by then I was only going to be 94, so I still had almost 2 thirds of my life to live. No I was far too young to die, and after all that's what cancer does, it kills people… doesn't it?

I don't know if cancer is the worst ailment to be diagnosed with; I don't know if there is a 'worst' illness category. Heart disease must be bloody awful to deal with too, and perhaps more paranoia inductive. If I had been told there was something seriously wrong with my heart I would imagine that I would be scared to move in case I wore it out. It's that 'you only have one' feeling.

MS, Parkinson's, HIV, Motor Neurone… there are so many diseases that cripple and debilitate the body and mess with the mind; and no doubt there are others that I have not yet heard of. Yet cancer is still the one that people are scared to talk about, still it is called The Big C as though saying the word 'cancer' aloud is the medical equivalent of saying 'Macbeth' in a theatre; as though the mere mention of the word will bring death knocking on the speaker's door. One in three people will, at some stage of their lives, be diagnosed with some form of cancer. But it is not the instant death sentence it once was; today's technology and medical breakthroughs mean that many people who face cancer will pull through, and will go on to live normal, healthy, if somewhat altered, lives.

So why didn't I call this book 'Living with Cancer', or give it some other similar title that would make it perfectly clear what this book is about? Jim Dancer is a term for cancer used in a book by Lee Dunne, a book called Goodbye to the Hill. This wonderful novel was written at a time when cancer was still, in most cases, a death sentence, a time when the mere mention of the word sent shivers down the spine. Lee is a friend of mine, an inspiration and a great support through those troubled times. So Jim Dancer... the name is in honour of him.

I saw a movie on TV the other day; one of those true life, guaranteed to make you cry, films about a young girl with cancer. The movie was called Lipstick, because her red lipstick made the heroine of the story feel good as she struggled to cope with the treatment that caused her to be sick and to loose her hair. But throughout the movie she kept meeting up with people she called 'angels', and I wondered if I should call this book 'Angels I have met along the way.' But I shook my head and told myself to quit being soppy.

My daughter, Melissa, was telling me the other day that during a discussion with her work colleagues someone commented that it seems as though many more people suffer from cancer today than they did in the past. My daughter rightly pointed out that this is due to the advancement of diagnostics, not that cancer it more prevalent than it once was.

In the past, as recently as 20 years ago, the diagnosis of cancer was often made when the disease had taken a firm hold, and there was little that could be done for the sufferer, other than invasive surgery or to offer palliative care. However, since then the development of CT, MRI and PET scanners have made it possible for doctors to find tumours long before they are inoperable and untreatable. These days the chances of not only surviving cancer but being cured of it completely, are much greater than they once were, not only because of diagnostics but also because of the breakthroughs in treatment that have been made by scientists who work tirelessly to find cures. Scientists who would be able to further their work a lot quicker if they had all the money they need to fund their research.

Everyone knows of Cancer Research, and of how this organisation has to raise funds in order to continue with their work. Who hasn't got a Cancer Research pen? Yet how many of us, until faced with cancer at a personal level, give even the cost of a cheap pen to the organisation? I have to hold my hand up and include myself here. Eventually tiring of all the different appeals that came to my door in one form or another, from varying charities asking for help, I decided a few years ago to choose 2 charities to give to on a regular basis, by direct debit. My method of deciding which charities to give to was simple; I chose The Red Cross, because they are on the front line of every disaster, no matter where it happens in the word. I chose The RSPCA, because animals cannot speak for themselves. And while I feel dreadful for having to admit it, Cancer Research didn't even enter my head. Why not? Because I believed then, and still believe now, that Cancer Research should not have to go cap in hand to the general public for funding. Cancer Research should be government funded, over and above the expense accounts of the politicians. And, of course there was the other aspect; the selfish thought that I wasn't going to get cancer.

I'm not about to go into a lengthy political rant about how the government wastes money that could be used for the betterment of the public. I don't know much about politics, and so couldn't make an educated statement about the fiscal abilities, or disabilities, of the government. I wouldn't dream of suggesting that politicians squeeze money out of their expense accounts like well dressed benefits cheats when this money would be put to better use in the hands of the people dedicated to finding cures for ills. But I do think it is very sad that people are still dying because Cancer Research, and other such life saving charities, needs funding that they have to ask the public to provide while politicians take second homes, top of the range cars and 5* hotels for granted and drain public funds to pay for the upkeep of luxurious lifestyles. Greedy, self-serving politicians are claiming millions that could be better used to look for a cure for many ailments while researchers have to beg the public for help.

A friend sent me this joke the other day, which just about sums up the sentiment of greedy politicians.

One day a florist goes to a barber for a haircut. After the cut he asked about his bill and the barber replies, 'I cannot accept money from you. I'm doing community service this week.' The florist was pleased and left the shop.

When the barber goes to open his shop the next morning there is a 'thank you' card and a dozen roses waiting for him at his door.

Later, a cop comes in for a haircut, and when he tries to pay his bill, the barber again replies, 'I cannot accept money from you. I'm doing community service this week.' The cop is happy and leaves the shop.

The next morning when the barber goes to open up there is a 'thank you' card and a dozen donuts waiting for him at his door.

Later that day, a college professor comes in for a haircut, and when he tries to pay his bill, the barber again replies, 'I cannot accept money from you, I'm doing community service this week.' The professor is very happy and leaves the shop.

The next morning when the barber opens his shop, there is a 'thank you' card and a dozen different books, such as 'How to Improve Your Business' and 'Becoming More Successful.'

Then, a Member of Parliament comes in for a haircut, and when he goes to pay his bill the barber again replies, 'I cannot accept money from you. I'm doing community service this week.' The Member of Parliament is very happy and leaves the shop.

The next morning when the barber goes to open up, there are a dozen Members of Parliament lined up waiting for a free haircut.

This may be intended as a joke, but like all the best jokes, it's based on reality.

Since writing the above the scandal of the expenses claimed by politicians has become headline news; we now know exactly how the politicians drain resources, how greedy they can be and how much the taxpayer has to fork out to cover expenses such as second homes.

The first time cancer was mentioned to me at a personal level was some 5 years ago. 2 years previous to this time I had a cyst removed from an ovary, and as the pain I was suffering this time was similar to the pain I had known from the invasion of the cyst, I had assumed that I had yet another piece of fruit attached to my inner workings.

I say a 'piece of fruit' because this is one of the measures used by educated medical people to describe the size of cysts and tumours. Men and women who have gone to the trouble of learning words like 'abdominoperineal' and 'zygomaticotemoral' (that's the a-z version), fail miserably when they attempt to illustrate the volume of cysts and tumours in anything other than the measurement of fruit and balls. My cyst had been the size of a large plum, and I have known other people to have cysts the size of grapes, oranges, grapefruits and, most unfortunately, melons. There is also the 'chocolate' cyst. This has nothing to do with a Terry's Chocolate Orange, but is a way of describing the appearance of a cyst that is full of dark blood, giving it the look of chocolate. All I can say to that is; yuck!

The alternative to fruit as a measurement for cysts and tumours is a load of balls (I said 'balls' not bollocks), which is not too bad if it's a squash ball, worse if it's a tennis ball, downright unlucky if the size of a rugby ball.

I can only assume that the use of fruit and balls to describe the size of cysts and tumours is to make it easier for the layperson to put the proportion of the growth into perspective. After all, a 5 centimetre cyst begs the questions; 5 centimetres in length? Circumference? Width? I suppose it has to make the Doctors' lives easier to describe the size in easily imagined everyday items.

As my first cyst had been the size of a plum; somewhere between a squash ball and a tennis ball, I assumed that this new cyst was considerably larger, perhaps even of cantaloupe proportions, going by the concerned expression on the consultant's face as she perched on the side of my hospital bed the day after she had performed a laparoscope; a small camera inserted through a very small cut just below the belly button, under general anaesthetic. She looked really worried; a frown etched her forehead with an '*I so pity you*' look that I didn't particularly like, or need, from a gynaecologist, or any doctor.

'It's not cancer,' she told me, and the look on her face changed slightly to one that said, '*I'm sure you'll be relieved to hear that.*' Yes I was relieved to hear that but, as I told the consultant.

'I hadn't thought for a moment that it was,' I said, and the end of the sentence rose in startled pitch, almost giving me an Australian accent. The thought of cancer had never entered my head. I had simply thought it was yet another cyst; cancer was something that old people got... wasn't it? And while I had not faced the prospect of another painful operation with anything approaching glee, I certainly hadn't thought that the pain I was suffering was life threatening or potentially incurable. A few days in hospital, a tiny scar... nothing *too* traumatic. Although, going by the way she was talking, the gynaecologist *had* suspected that it was cancer prior to performing a laparoscope to take a look inside. These days the slightest little pain anywhere in my body makes me paranoid that it could be cancer, but back then, even though I had been suffering horrendous pain, I hadn't thought about cancer for a moment.

'So is it a big one?' I asked, reverting back to my cyst theory, which was obviously correct, as it was not cancer. Mrs Sharon looked confused.

'Is what a big one?' She asked.

'The cyst,' I reminded her.

'What cyst?' She looked totally bewildered now.

'The cyst on my ovary,' I explained, wondering why I had to guide her to her diagnosis.

'There is no cyst on your ovary,' Mrs Sharon finally caught up with the conversation and cottoned on to my train of thought. 'You have endometriosis,' she explained.

Although, to be honest, that really wasn't any form of explanation; it was just a big word that got itself tied all around my tongue when I tried to repeat it. Mrs Sharon repeated the word for me, but it was days before I finally managed to say it without stammering. In case you are struggling to pronounce the word; phonetically it is *end~o~meat~ree~o~sis*.

Mrs Sharon explained what endometriosis was, and that because it was particularly bad in my case there was no option other than to remove my womb, and everything attached to it; my ovaries, cervix and any connecting pipe-work had to go. Endometriosis is a particularly icky condition, one that I won't go into here, just in case you are eating. There's a whole section on the subject on Wikipedia if you really need to know more. Failing that, I am sure some celebrity has written a book about it at some stage.

I lay in bed, listening to her tell me that she needed to perform extensive surgery on me, with growing dread of the pain this was going to produce for me. A friend of my mother's had to go through a hysterectomy a few years before, and she was in agony for weeks afterwards, even after they sent her home to recover. Mrs Sharon saw the fear and worry in my expression and touched my hand gently.

'We can arrange counselling for you,' she told me. But I really couldn't see how talking about the pain was going to be any help at all. 'Many women find it difficult to cope with losing their womb,' she added, and again I realised that our thoughts were on different tracks. I told her I was not concerned about losing my womb, but that I was concerned about the level of pain I was going to go through afterwards. She assured me that modern pain relief would be provided and that I would be made as comfortable as possible after the operation. I didn't ask what would happen if I didn't have the operation; this was information I didn't need. All I needed to know what that the pain I had been suffering recently would be gone once I had recovered from the surgery.

While my hysterectomy was *not* associated with cancer, for many women this is exactly why they have to undergo this major surgery. And I know that, for many women, this is a very traumatic operation for more reasons than the pain that was my main concern at the time. It is not only 'women of a certain age' who have to go under the surgeon's knife in this way, but also young women, some of who have yet to have children of their own, or women who had hoped to add to the family they already have. I can only imagine how heartbreaking it must be to loose your womb when it was still your intention to have children, and it is for such women that counselling is important.

As I began to write this, the news was full of Jade Goody's funeral. Jade was one such young mother who had to undergo a hysterectomy because of cancer of the cervix. But in Jade's case it was too little too late. She had been told a long time ago that she needed to do something about the cells the doctors found during a smear test. Instead she chose to go into the Big Brother house and put some more money into the bank. They (the media) say that she left a legacy that will save the lives of other young girls who may be tempted to ignore the early warning signs as Jade herself did. They say that Jade's death was not in vain; that because of her young women all over the country are going for smear tests. Perhaps this is the case, but still, it is a crying shame that she is now dead at the age of 27. Yes, she has left a lot of money for her young sons, but which one of them would not give it all away for a few more years with their mother?

Perhaps I am cynical, but I can't help wondering if all the media hype surrounding Jade Goody had less to do with caring about her and more to do with making money out of her tragic circumstances. Jade may have made money for her sons, so that they could live comfortably when she was gone, but how much more did the media make from her?

She was barely cold in her grave before a book was released in her name; the diary of her death; ghost writing takes on a whole new meaning as I am sure that this book will have been put together by a professional writer who is still very much alive, from sketchy diary entries made by Jade and her mother. No doubt this will sell in hundreds of thousands; although, I find it difficult to believe that Jade and her mother wrote the whole diary. It seems that the public can't get enough of suffering, so long as it's happening to someone else. Am I the only one who feels just a little sick at the notion of how much money the media have made on the back of Jade's misery? And am I the only one who finds it more than a touch ironic that the TV channel that followed Jade around is called the Living channel? OK magazine were so keen to get their copies sold that they even brought out the 'in memory' edition *before* Jade died.

But this is classic 'it won't happen to me' way of thinking. Even though cancer happens to one in three of us, we all feel that it will happen to someone else, that we are invincible, that we are going to live forever, that we can put off whatever treatment there is because we are busy with our lives and don't want to be bothered with our deaths, not yet, not until we are ready, and even then we are all going to die peacefully in our sleep. Did anyone tell Jade that she would die if she ignored the early warnings? It's hard to believe that anyone would not go for treatment if they really believed they would die without it.

In my case the hysterectomy I was facing was not to save my life, not at that point, it was merely to get rid of what was causing excruciating pain; at least, I think it wasn't to save my life, but I'm not entirely sure if endometrioses could be a life-threatening problem. But going through the proposed operation was going to put me through more pain, although only in the short term, yet I was still scared stiff at the prospect.

I explained to Mrs Sharon that I was not remotely concerned about losing my uterus. After all, my youngest son was in his late 20s by that stage and to find myself in a position where my womb was being used again would have been downright embarrassing for my children. No, that's not what was bothering me. What was bothering me was the prospect of pain. My pain threshold was then, and is now, practically non-existent; a strong wind can make me say 'ouch'.

Mrs Sharon again promised me that pain relief was much better now than it was when Bridie, Mum's friend, had her operation, and that the drugs *would* work, in spite of that dreadful, morose song by The Verve that stated otherwise.

And so a date was arranged for me to go into hospital to have a hysterectomy, including various pipes and other bits and pieces that needed to come out too. Was I scared? No, I was not scared; I was bloody terrified and wanted to run away.

Apparently wanting to run away when faced with any traumatic situation is perfectly normal; it's all part of the 'fight or flee' instinct that everyone goes through when faced with difficult situations.

I was given a date to check in to the hospital, the date was the day before the planned operation; I assume they didn't trust me to fast properly if they let me stay at home until the following day. Not that I could have eaten a thing; terror does that to me; it completely closes my throat so that no food will go down (Oh the irony).

Tom brought me to the hospital, and stayed with me while the nurse checked me in, but eventually he had to go, leaving me to pace up and down the ward when I wasn't walking up and down the corridors to the front door to smoke. I didn't sleep much that night; I don't believe anyone sleeps much in hospital unless they are deaf or have the good sense to bring earplugs into hospital with them, as I did on future occasions when I had to be admitted. All night doors banged, hinges squeaked, loud whispers muttered in the distance and eventually the dawn broke to herald the day, the day of the dreaded operation.

On the morning of the operation I was given a gown to wear that had 'hospital use only' printed all over it in bright shades of red, yellow, green and blue. I couldn't help wondering; if it were not for this print would I be tempted to take it home with me for future special occasions? I still wonder what bright spark decided it necessary to print those words all over the gowns, and how much extra it cost for the printed ones as against the plain ones. If I had been given a plain gown would I have smuggled it out of the hospital in my case as though it were a fluffy robe from a 5* hotel? Not that I steal gowns from 5* hotels; for one thing I have never stayed at a 5* hotel and for another I am no thief. Perhaps the primary colours were meant to have some sort of psychological 'happy' effect... that didn't work. Whatever the reason for the print, it simply struck me as a dreadful waste of money when the NHS is constantly struggling for funds.

Some people like the feeling of going to sleep under general anaesthetic. I don't; I hate that feeling of losing control over my entire being as the warmth spreads up my arm. Most people say that when they come to from an operation that they can't feel any pain; but in my case I now know to beg the anaesthetist, prior to any procedure, to give me as much as possible of any drug they have that may numb the pain.

In the case of the hysterectomy operation I woke up in the recovery room feeling as though I had been stabbed, which I had been. Actually, I had been more than stabbed. I had been sliced open, had a lot of my internal bits and pieces cut away, and had been stapled back together. But if I had imagined I would wake from the op without any pain I was so wrong. The pain was intense, so intense that it felt as though no anaesthetic whatsoever had been used.

What had I been thinking prior to the op? I had managed to convince myself that I wouldn't feel a thing; that the drugs would take away every last vestige of pain that I could possibly have felt? I had assumed that modern surgery techniques meant that nobody felt *any* pain after extensive surgery, and I blame TV for that! In Holby, people come to after heart surgery and other such operations looking as though they are in no pain whatsoever, and as everyone knows, TV is a representation of real life.

I don't mean to scare anyone here, but surgery *is* painful. Then again, I'm probably the only fool in the world to think otherwise.

Eventually they got the pain under control, and gave me a button to press so that I could administer morphine to myself. This made me feel a lot better; the notion that I could press the green button and morphine would course through my veins helped with the pain enormously and I pressed it every couple of seconds. It was much later that I found out that the pump only allows a certain amount of morphine through, and that if it had provided opiates with every press of the green button I would probably have died of an overdose!

Of course, any extensive surgery *is* painful, and Holby City/Casualty/ER are *not* representations of reality. The people who come through invasive surgery on TV are only actors and in real life pain relief can only offer a certain amount of respite because pain is really quite important as an indication of what is going on with the body.

Without pain we would not know when we have serious injury and could be walking around with broken limbs. Without pain we would have no measure of our recuperation process and would have no idea whether or not we are getting better. Pain is an essential evaluation tool that allows doctors to assess what is going on in our bodies... but I still don't like it. When I pressed the button on the morphine pump it was as though I was tapping out some maniacal Morse code to the god Morpheus, begging him to come and take away my pain. I only stopped short of offering a sacrifice.

When the effects of the anaesthetic eventually began to diminish, and something akin to lucidity was slowly coming back to me, I realised that other parts of my body were affected by the operation too, because whatever way I tried to move, I was using my stomach muscles in some small way, muscles that were protesting hugely at being used for anything more than gentle breathing. And coughing… well, that was reduced to a gentle 'ahem' sound, as though I were very politely trying to get someone's attention in a library. And for the first time in my life, the last thing I wanted to do was to smoke.

I first started smoking when I was 11 years old, and although I had given up several times, seldom for longer than a few hours, I had no desire whatsoever to smoke after my hysterectomy. Before the operation I had dashed outside the hospital for one last frantic ciggie. Like any smoker, I believed this would help to calm my nerves. Cigarettes do *not* calm the nerves… this is just a myth, probably started by tobacco companies, the legal drug pushers in my opinion. I was still a gibbering wreck as I made the long walk to the operating theatre with my pillow tucked under my arm, my last cigarette having done nothing whatsoever to calm my jittery nerves. And after the operation, well, I knew I would *never* smoke again.

Another woman, in hospital at the same time as myself and having the same operation preformed on the same day, came to my bedside the following day to ask if I wanted to go outside for a smoke.

'*Are you mad? Are you completely off your head? Go away you crazy woman.*' I screamed at her in my mind, while uttering a polite 'No thanks, I think I have given up smoking now.' I watched her shuffle off, knowing that she had about 200 yards to cover in order to get to the front door of the hospital before she would be able to smoke, and knowing that once she did so she would no doubt cough. The thought made me shudder, the shudder hurt my tummy, and I was absolutely *certain* that I would never smoke again. I didn't need patches, gum or pills. Pain was enough for me to kick the habit for good.

She wasn't alone though; there were several other women who regularly made the arduous journey to the front door of the hospital for their fix. After every meal they would gather at the door to the ward and shuffle off down the corridor, some wheeling stands that held necessary fluids and anti-biotics, until they reached an area where they could light up without anyone wagging a finger at them and saying 'tut-tut'. The pathetic little troupe of hardened smokers made me shake my head in wonder that anyone could be so desperate for a cigarette that they could put themselves through such torture in order to fill their lungs and their bloodstreams with tobacco.

Tobacco is a terrible drug that grips the user like no narcotic can. If tobacco were to be introduced into society today, it would be banned, and rightly so. Tobacco kills more people every year than heroin and crack cocaine, and yet it is available at the supermarket. Why? Because the government receive a massive amount of revenue from tobacco sales, that would be missed from the budget if the deadly substance were to be banned. Without the revenue from tobacco the politicians would have to drive Fiestas and stay at Mrs Jackson's B&B when the party conference is taking place. Am I ranting about politicians again?

Anyway, I had given up smoking by the time I was allowed home later that week, and family and friends were respectful of this, going out into the back yard to smoke when the need gripped them. Strangely, this made me feel like a social pariah; the only other people I know who do not smoke are my youngest son and his wife. Unfortunately they lived hundreds of miles away at the time, so while everyone else was out in the back yard, enjoying the spring sunshine and one another's company, I spent most of my time alone in the smoke free environment that my home had become.

Eventually I started smoking again. I got stressed out over something so important that I can't remember for the life of me what it was and I just had one cigarette. Then I got stressed out over something else equally unimportant and it was a slippery slope until I was, once again, smoking like the proverbial trooper.

Recovery from the hysterectomy was slow. A friend of mine had the same operation done a week after me, and she was running in the marathon a few weeks later while I was still nearly crying in pain every time I tried to stand up. Ok, so she wasn't *actually* running in the marathon, but she *was* out walking her dogs and, to my shame, visiting me to see if I needed anything doing.

Chapter Two – Not well

For the next couple of years I didn't feel too well. I can't really explain what I mean by that other than it was as though I were coming down with something that never happened, a cold hiding in the background that never broke out. Now and then I would go to the doctor, the doctor would carry out blood tests etc, but they couldn't find anything of any significance other than a slightly raised white blood cell count. I had no appetite, and my body learned how to live on small amounts of food. I visited the doctor regularly as time went on, but because they could find nothing wrong with me I began to suspect I was a hypochondriac. I think they suspected I was a hypochondriac too, going by the way they looked at me, if that's not just me being paranoid.

Every so often blood tests would try to determine the cause of my feeling ill. But other than a high white cell count, there was nothing significant to say that there was anything in particular wrong with me. Every time they said my white cell count was high the thought occurred to me that this is indicative of cancer. But because the doctors didn't mention this fact I assumed (to assume is to make and ass out of u and me [ass-u-me]) that they knew that this could not be the case, that my white cell count was not high enough to indicate cancer. Only a true hypochondriac would push this matter, and I wasn't one, I genuinely didn't feel well.

During this time my cousin, Suzanne, found out that she had cancer, a huge tumour that was stuck to several internal organs, including her lungs. She was only in her early 50s, had never smoked, seldom drank and although she had been a true hypochondriac for most of her life this was real and this devastated her.

Sue was a human Google, and sometimes even better than Google. I used to call her our female Stephen Fry. Although to be fair, she was probably smarter and more knowledgeable than Stephen. There is no search engine where you can 'dum de, dum dum dum' to find out what a particular tune is. But Sue would tell you not only the name of the tune but who wrote it, when it was published and any other interesting facts that you may like to know. She was a super brain who could answer any question that was not mathematical (Like me, Sue had an aversion to maths that we both agreed was a form of dyslexia.). Why would any God make a woman like Sue and then decide to wipe her out? It didn't make sense to me then and it still doesn't now.

Yet, in spite of her intelligence and knowledge she declined the offer of chemotherapy that could have given her a much longer life than the three years that she was to have. Sue didn't want to lose her hair, and no amount of coaxing and cajoling would shift her decision once it was made.

I tried to talk her into having the treatment by appealing to her sense of fun.

'You can have a different wig for every day of the week if you like,' I told her, but she was having none of it. If her time had come, then amen meant 'so be it' to Suzanne.

So, while I was feeling a bit off colour, it was nothing to what Sue was suffering, and so I put my vague illness to the back of my mind. Sue died in the January of 2006. By the time she died my malady situation had got no worse, but no better. I wasn't ill; I was just unwell… if that makes sense.

I was on a bit of a high during the latter part of that year. Although, sadly, Sue had not lived to see my book on the shelves, Gill & Macmillan published my memoir, The Mun, in Ireland that September. It was launched by several radio interviews, I had a 2 page spread in the Sunday World (one of Ireland's biggest selling Sunday papers) and I was on top of the world. Not the literary world, but still, having my book published was a great achievement and I didn't need to sell millions of copies in order to have my writing ability recognised. That my book was on the shelves, published by a respected publishing house, was enough for me. There it was on Amazon, and on the shelves of every Dublin bookstore. It would have been a bonus if the book had made me a fortune, but then it was hardly Harry Potter.

I still went to the doctor occasionally, complaining of not feeling well, my appetite was practically non-existent by this stage, but it wasn't until November 2006 that I developed a dreadful throat infection. So I was given a course of antibiotics, and by Christmas the infection was gone.

A couple of glands had come up on my neck with the throat infection, but as everyone knows this is perfectly normal with a throat infection, so it didn't worry me unduly. However, after Christmas one of the glands, the one on the right side of my neck, stayed up, and grew to about the size of a squash ball (the balls thing works). It wasn't painful; I didn't feel any more ill than I had over the past couple of years, so I put off going to the doctor yet again. I was sure by this stage that I was being looked upon as some sort of malingering hypochondriac who was desperate for some terrible disease to be found. This was far from the truth; I wanted to be told that there was *nothing* wrong with me; I wanted to know this for sure.

My eldest son, Owen, called to visit one night, and as he was leaving he frowned at my neck.

'You want to get that looked at Mum,' he told me. And perhaps that was why I made an appointment to see Dr Fola, a new doctor at our surgery who I had not seen before. Dr Fola is not her real name. She is African, and apparently her real name is difficult to pronounce, so she goes by the name of Fola to make life easy for us Europeans.

She gave me a thorough examination, checking not only my throat but also under my armpits, and around my groin area; I was way too ignorant to ask why but she obviously knew what she was doing and I was impressed that she was being so methodical. She sent me away with a prescription for a course of antibiotic tablets, telling me to go back to see her if the gland did not go down. It didn't go down, so two weeks later I had another consultation with her that led to another course of antibiotic tablets, which I duly collected from the chemist's on my way home. I had only been home a few minutes when the phone rang. I was surprised to hear Dr Fola's voice on the line; as we all know it's a rare day when a doctor rings a patient at home, unless you are a celebrity being treated privately.

'I've been thinking, and while I still want you to take the antibiotics I would like you to see a specialist with that gland,' she told me. 'You should hear from them within the next couple of weeks,' she added. And while a better informed person may have thought '2 week rule' and gone into a state of panic from the implications of that thought, I was merely honoured that she cared enough about my welfare to get me seen so quickly. How ignorant was I?

A week later I attended Lancaster hospital for an appointment with Miss Ahmed, a very beautiful gentle lady with a caring manner. She had a look at the back of my throat and decided that it would be best if my right tonsil came out.

Ah, so that's what the problem was... a dodgy tonsil. That made sense. As a child I was plagued by sore throats and was to have my tonsils out when I was ten years old; but my parents had decided to move to Ireland at the same time, and my operation never happened. Obviously time had caught up with me and it was now quite important that the offending tonsil be removed.

Easy… after having a hysterectomy, a tonsillectomy, singular at that, was going to be a piece of cake. Ok, I didn't *want* to be in hospital, not being a true hypochondriac, but as the procedure couldn't be done at home, I bit the bullet again and checked in to the hospital for the minor operation.

It wasn't too bad as operations go. I was in and out within a couple of days. As soon as I could prove I was fit to leave, the criteria being the consumption of a couple of slices of toast, I was allowed to go home. I was given an appointment to see Miss Ahmed a couple of weeks later to make sure that the tonsil area had healed properly and was sent home to recover.

But I didn't recover, not properly, and a couple of days later my sore throat got worse, and when I looked at the back of my throat in the mirror it seemed to have a strange green tint to it. The fact that I was trying to smoke cannot have been helping the situation. My husband was outside in the back street, and I thought I should let him have a look too.

'Do you think my throat looks ok?' I asked him, opening my mouth wide so that he could take a look inside. He reeled back, recoiling with jazz hands, and suggested that I call a doctor. But this was a bank holiday Monday, so I couldn't go to the doctors' surgery. At this time the NHS ran a wonderful help-line where trained medical staff were on hand to offer advice when it is not possible to get to the doctor; so I called 0845 46 47 and spoke to a nurse who assured me that green was not the normal colour for my throat to be. She arranged for a doctor to visit and once again I was given a strong course of antibiotics. The doctor who visited told me I had simply been unlucky, that this happened to some people who had tonsils out, and I assumed that this was what people meant when they said it was more dangerous to have tonsils out in adulthood than as a child. There I go with my assumptions again.

I didn't tell the doctor that I had been smoking; I didn't need to tell her this to know that she was going to frown and tell me that she would not recommend smoking after having a tonsil out. Of course she would not recommend smoking with an open throat wound; I knew that anyone who smoked after having tonsils out was beyond mad, but that didn't stop me wanting to.

Now I know that she could *smell* the smoke from me. Of course she could; in just the same way that I can smell smoke on someone at a hundred paces these days. Anyone who doesn't smoke can smell it on someone who has been at the tobacco. Mints, mouth fresheners… don't kid yourself, if you have been smoking and you're not supposed to, then to anyone who doesn't smoke you absolutely stink. It makes me cringe now to think that I smelled like that for so many years. The public information broadcasts are not exaggerating; smokers really do smell like mucky ashtrays to non-smokers.

My throat got better, and a few days later I went off for my appointment with Miss Ahmed so that she could tell me everything was fine and that she didn't need to see me again. My throat was clear, I was able to smoke again without any discomfort (not that I would be telling Miss Ahmed this), and the gland in my neck seemed a lot smaller than it had been before the tonsil had been removed. It wasn't totally gone, but it was obviously getting smaller and would eventually be gone altogether, or so I assumed.

'We didn't find anything in the tonsil that we removed,' Miss Ahmed informed me, and I probably nodded. I certainly didn't panic when she said this. I didn't ask what it was that she had *expected* to find. Not finding 'anything' was good… wasn't it? Let's not push the issue. 'I would like to remove that gland.' She went on to say.

Miss Ahmed explained that as the gland had not gone down completely, she would like to remove it surgically, and I didn't ask why. I simply assumed that she knew what she was doing, and that if she thought the procedure was necessary then I would just have to go along with her decision; I wasn't particularly attached to any of my glands. And so the arrangements were made, and a few days later I was checking back into the same ward where I had been when my tonsil was removed.

Miss Ahmed had told me that when I came to I would have a drain attached to the wound, and that it would only be when this drain had stopped collecting fluid that I would be able to go home. The drain was a little, plastic bottle, about 2 inches in depth, which concertinaed in the middle. A tube was attached to the top of the little bottle, the end of which was under my skin, just above my right shoulder. The pain from the operation wasn't too bad, and the little plastic bottle didn't bother me too much. When it came to having the drain removed so that I could go home I was relieved that it had all gone well, and that the annoying gland had finally gone.

Miss Ahmed came to see me before I went home; she sat on the side of the bed and explained that the operation had gone well. She screwed her nose up a bit and said.

'The gland was rather nasty.' So obviously her decision to remove it had been a good one. 'You did very well,' she told me, patting the back of my hand. I though she had done even better; and I told her so.

I had seen the scar in the mirror, and I was mightily impressed with her needlework. Although the operation had only been performed three days earlier, already it was plain to see that the scar would be barely noticeable once it was properly healed. An appointment was made for me to return to her clinic a couple of weeks later, I assumed to have the stitches removed and to see her for the last time.

In case you haven't noticed, I was assuming an awful lot throughout this period of my life. Looking back now it was almost as though I had been blindfolded, had earmuffs in place and was singing la, la, la. I wasn't hearing anything to make me worry, and I wasn't seeing anything that concerned me unduly. I was simply allowing myself to be led through a series of procedures that I trusted the professionals to perform as necessary, without ever asking *why* these procedures were necessary.

Miss Ahmed shared her clinic with Mr Kochar, and it was Mr Kochar that I saw when I went back to Lancaster hospital for my final check up. I could see how these two people worked so well together. Like Miss Ahmed, Mr Kochar had a gentle nature, and he looked at me with a caring expression on his face. He gently removed the stitches from my neck, and I didn't feel a thing.

I waited while he sat back down and looked at my file. Waiting for him to tell me that everything was fine and I could go home; there was no reason for me to go back to the hospital any more, not now that the offending gland had been properly dealt with. And I waited. Was he a slow reader?

Eventually Mr Kochar sighed; was it an involuntary sigh? Did he even realise he had done so? He looked at me and I could tell that he had to steel himself to look into my eyes.

'We found cancer in the gland that we took from your neck,' he told me, and I felt as though he had punched me in the stomach. But then I remembered, not all tumours are malignant.

'Was it malignant or benign?' I asked him. Ever optimistic, I expected him to tell me that the cancer had indeed been benign.

'All cancers are malignant,' Mr Kochar educated me. 'Tumours may be benign in that there are no cancerous cells contained in them, but cancer is always malignant,' he said, filling me in on a subject that I would rather have remained ignorant about.

'But Miss Ahmed managed to get it out,' I said to Mr Kochar, confident that the surgery had removed the malignant invader.

Mr Kochar explained that while Miss Ahmed had managed to remove the gland that had contained the cancer, the cells found there was secondary cancer, and that somewhere there was a primary cancer that had yet to be discovered.

Even as I write that here, I feel a little sick, my head feels dizzy and the memory of that day fills my mind with the same dread that it did then.

I have little recollection of the conversation that followed with Mr Kochar. Miss Ahmed came into the room and they both spoke to me about what was likely to happen next. But I didn't take in what they were telling me in any great detail; I *couldn't* take I their words because my mind was busy trying to deal with the fact that cancer had been found in my neck and I was about to die. My head shot up my arse when Mr Kochar told me that cancer had been found in the gland that had been removed, and it's difficult to hear *anything* while using bum cheeks as earmuffs.

Another operation was necessary, to remove the lymph nodes in the right side of my neck. I had asked Miss Ahmed if she would be performing this operation, but she told me that she didn't have the necessary expertise to carry this one out, and I would be going to Preston, to see a Mr Small, an appointment would be sent out in the post to confirm this.

I didn't want to see Mr Small, whoever he was. I wanted Miss Ahmed to do the operation; I wanted it to be done at Lancaster, not Preston. Lancaster hospital is a nice little hospital, whereas Preston was a big, scary place, in my head anyway.

I had to decide whether or not to tell the children what was going on. They all knew about the operations I had so far, and they had been as worried as I had been about the potential outcome. In other words, they had not been worried at all. Until the day when I was told about the cancer cells being found in the gland that had been removed, nobody had mentioned cancer at all, so apart from having a couple of minor operations to remove unwanted parts, there hadn't been *anything* to worry about.

When I say 'children'… my kids were all in their thirties, so it's not as though I needed to find any picture books to explain things to them, they were all more than capable of understanding what was going on. But I knew that as soon as I told them that cancer cells had been found in the gland they were going to worry, and I didn't want them to have a moment's worry, not about me, not about anything. As a mother, I wanted my children to have worry-free lives, and I didn't want to be responsible for giving them any sleepless nights.

But the alternative to telling them the truth was lying to them, and covering up whatever was going to happen. While I considered this, I also knew that they were going to suspect something was seriously wrong when I told them I had to have yet another operation. All they had to do was Google the matter and they were likely to come up with the knowledge that I was not being entirely honest with them.

So I decided not to lie, but nor was I going to scare the living daylights out of them by letting them know how scared I was. So I told them that cancer had been found in the gland in my neck, and that this gland had been successfully removed. I told them that the other glands were going to be removed to be on the safe side. I didn't actually tell them that there was nothing to worry about, or that the next operation was nothing more than a precautionary measure. But I know that's the impression I gave. I wasn't trying to be glib about what was happening, but nor did I want to worry the children unduly. Besides, if I admitted my fears to my children, I would be admitting them to myself.

Nor did I want to worry my parents.

My parents were both in their eighties by this stage, and were from an era where nobody lived through cancer; a time when Jim Dancer was still spoken of in hushed tones, in reverence of the disease that surely killed anyone it grew in. I didn't want to tell lies to my parents, but I knew I had to do so, for as long as possible. They knew about the operations I already had, and they would have to know about the operation that would be happening sometime soon, but the word 'cancer' had never been mentioned, and so long as this word remained unspoken, they would not have to worry about their only child dying before them. Not that I planned on dying, but I knew that this would be their worry if I told them that cancer had been found, and I couldn't bear the idea of them making themselves ill with worry.

Later that night I watched TV in an automated way because I didn't know what else to do with my evening, but I wasn't taking it in or enjoying it. Desperate Housewives is one of my favourite TV shows, and it was on that night, so I flicked over to the channel it was showing on. And by one of those dreadful coincidences in life, it was the episode where Lynette was told she had cancer. I remember thinking how wonderful it must be for the outcome of cancer to be in the hands of a team of writers.

I got my first appointment to see Mr Small in early May. As I expected, Preston hospital was huge, even bigger than it had been in my imagination. It is made up of many different buildings, designed by many different architects; the overall affect being that it more resembles a small town than a singular hospital. Inside the main doors it was like walking into an airport concourse; there were shops, restaurants and even a beauty salon so that anyone needing that particular kind of pick-me-up didn't have to leave the hospital to have their hair or nails done.

After walking along corridors, going down in lifts, going up and down stairs and trawling even more corridors, we finally came to the Ear, Nose and Throat (ENT) department and discovered that we could have parked just outside and that the long walk from the main entrance had been a waste of energy.

The waiting room was packed; a small TV in the corner was trying to entertain the masses with reruns of Bargain Hunt that nobody really wanted to watch. Besides, the reception was so bad that it was difficult to understand what the presenters were saying in between the hissing and crackling. I'm sure if I had been receiving private treatment the TV would have been a huge flat screen job with 2000 channels. But this was the NHS, and TV was not a priority.

Being a patient patient is recommended while waiting in an NHS waiting room. Anyone who expects to be seen at the allotted time should make sure that they get the first appointment of the day, otherwise, be prepared to wait.

One man was getting very angry because more than an hour had passed since his wife's allotted appointment time, and every so often he would go up to the reception desk and complain loudly, much to the embarrassment of his wife, who was more than happy to wait her turn like everyone else.

The problem arises because of over booking; which you may think is an inefficient way of dealing with things. And you would probably be right, but what else can they do? How would you feel if you were told 'Sorry, we can't see you next week because we are fully booked.'? They often *are* fully booked, and I'm sure that's not just Preston, but because people have to be seen they overbook, the doctors work longer than they are supposed to, but in the end everyone who needs to be seen gets a turn. And in my experience the appointments are never hurried. There is no point in complaining. OK, if you think you may have been overlooked, by all means ask at the reception desk, but complaining will get you nowhere.

While sitting waiting I heard a sound that I had not heard for a long time; it was the sound of someone speaking with the assistance of one of those electronic devices that people use when their larynx no longer works, usually because of surgery associated with cancer. It is known as an artificial larynx... no surprises there.

Sometimes we know we shouldn't be amused, and try really hard not to laugh, and for me this was one of those times. Why? Because it wasn't just one person speaking with one of these devices, it was two people having a conversation, and they both sounded identical. From where I sat, around the corner from the unseen conversationalists, it sounded like a Dalek invasion.

I know, I know... I really should not have been thinking that way. And I wonder if it may have been my way of dealing with the dread of ending up with one of those machines myself.

I took an instant liking to Mr Small, a straight speaking Scot, in spite of the fact that the first thing he did was to shove a camera up my nose.

Anyone suspected of having cancer of the head and neck is likely to have a camera shoved up their nose at some time; in my case this was every time I visited Preston hospital from that day forward. Of course it is not a large Nikon, of the variety worn by Japanese tourists while doing the rounds of European landmarks. The nose camera is a long, thin tube that is passed through a nostril and down the throat so that the consultant can have a good look to see what it going on down there. In my case this proved to be nothing apparent.

Before inserting the camera Mr Small sprayed some liquid up my nostrils, some kind of local anaesthesia to make sure the experience is not a painful one. That said, having a camera shoved up the nostril, however gently, and with whatever local anaesthesia, is never going to be a pleasant experience. But at worst I can only call it 'uncomfortable'. It makes the eyes water a bit, but it doesn't hurt.

He didn't see anything to concern him. There was nothing apparent in my throat to alarm him in any way. But still...

'I'm going to make arrangements for you to come in to have lymph glands removed from the right side of your neck,' he told me, and I refrained from quipping about that being good, that it would be a shame to get the wrong side.

Mr Small went on to explain that the cancer cells were secondary, and that the lymph glands had acted as a safety net, catching the cells before they could go to other areas. He told me that he would take out as many as possible, and then he told me that I might have to go through some radiotherapy afterwards to make sure they got all of the bad cells.

From what he told me it sounded as though this operation was going to be similar to the one that Miss Ahmed had carried out to remove the big gland. So, regarding the operation itself, I wasn't too worried. But what I was worried about was the cancer... where the hell was it?

Prior to the operation Mr Small arranged for a PET scan to be carried out to see if any active cells could be found. A PET scan is where radioactive sugar is injected into the bloodstream. It is not painful or uncomfortable in any way. The worst part of a PET scan is boredom, waiting an hour for the sugar to travel through the body before the scan itself can be done; the scan takes about 20 minutes, and again is not at all painful or uncomfortable. Because my scan was looking for active cells in the head and neck area I wasn't even allowed to read to pass the time, as reading uses up muscles in the eyes and could have given a false reading.

This scan was done on a Friday, in a new area of the hospital that looked more like a private hospital than a department of the NHS. A large flat screen TV, complete with cable channels, was fixed to the wall, the chairs were large, plush, leather armchairs, and in the corner there was a machine where free drinks were available to anyone who needed to be there, patients and their companions.

Because I had to fast all day in preparation for the scan, by the time it was over I was seriously hungry. So on the way home we stopped at a little country pub and had big, crusty sandwiches. I ordered Cajun chicken, and although I was surprised to find it was served cold, I was hungry, so I ate it.

It was Sunday before the pain in my stomach started, and by Monday it was so bad that I felt as though my belly could explode. I rang my local doctor's surgery and got an emergency appointment for that evening.

Of course, this was it, this was where the cancer was, it was in my stomach and the PET scan had obviously escalated the problem so that the huge tumour in my stomach had grown and multiplied over the weekend. Even though I had dreadful diarrhoea I was convinced that the pain was cancer and that I was going to die pretty soon if the pain was any sort of indication of life expectancy.

Dr Walker didn't laugh at my suggestion that this could be where the primary cancer was located, but I'm sure he wanted to. He was pretty sure that I either had a tummy bug, or that I had food poisoning. And as I had to admit that the pain had subsided somewhat since the onset of the diarrhoea it seemed that he was right.

'So where could it be?' I asked, desperate for some sort of an answer as to where my primary cancer was located.

'Somewhere in the head and neck region; most likely the throat area,' Dr Walker told me, and then he went on to explain that the cells that had been found, squamous cells, were only found in this area. 'The PET scan should be able to tell us more when the results come back,' he added, but he was wrong.

The PET scan didn't find *any* active cells, and where the primary source was located was still a mystery. But, just as a precaution, Mr Small decided to go ahead with the operation and I waited for the telephone call to tell me when I had to report to the hospital to have the procedure carried out.

'Friday 13th July,' Mr Small's secretary informed me when the phone call finally came.

Friday the 13th!

I'm not normally a superstitious person, but I wasn't at all keen on having the operation on that particular date. But then I told myself that if people died on the operating table on Friday 13th as a regular thing, surely this would have attracted media interest. It was not at all practical to shut down every operating theatre on this date.

I won't say I wasn't scared. I reckon it is perfectly obvious by now that I am something of a wimp when it comes to hospitals and operations. But at least I had already had this operation done once before, when Miss Ahmed had removed the nasty gland, so I had a fair idea of what I had to face. I had been through it once; I could get through it again.

But meanwhile, a trip to Dublin had been planned. My mum, my daughter Melissa, my granddaughter Jade, my friend Tracy and I had planned this trip before we knew I was going to need any surgery, and if anyone ever needed a holiday…

We flew out of Blackpool, and aged 33 this was to be my daughter's first ever flight. She was utterly terrified, and rediscovered Catholicism as the plane's wheels left the tarmac, blessing herself with the sure and certain knowledge that this action would ensure her place in Heaven if the plane were to come down in the middle of the Irish Sea. Every bump brought forth a whimper, every air pocket produced a small scream of terror, and the other passengers were kept entertained; any apprehension anyone else may have had kept at bay by her fear on the short journey.

It was a wonderful week and we filled every moment of every day with memories to last a lifetime and did enough shopping to call for an extra suitcase on the way home. I also found a new friend during that holiday.

On our way to Kilmainham Jail in a taxi that Thursday afternoon, we were heading up Dame Street when the taxi driver said: 'Would you look who's over there; it's only Lee Dunne himself.' And he pointed back down the road to where Lee was ambling along, looking in shop windows. (For anyone who has not heard of Lee, he is one of Ireland's most prolific writers, and holds the accolade of being Ireland's most banned writer. Many years ago I had read everything I could get my hands on by him, and was more than familiar with his work.) We stopped at traffic lights, and Lee was right there next to us on the pavement. I rolled down the window and asked if I could take his picture. 'Of course you can,' he replied with a smile, and politely posed for the picture. The lights changed, the taxi moved on, and it was to be another two years before I would see Lee again.

On our return from Dublin I found Lee's website and emailed him to thank him for letting me take his photograph. To my surprise he mailed back, so I mailed back, and soon we had swapped addresses, sent one another signed copies of our books and a firm friendship developed. It was some time later that I found out that Lee's beloved mother, Katie, had died from the very same cancer that I was about to start battling with.

The fun was over, the holiday a wonderful memory, and the future… well, that was the operation that I booked myself in for on the 12th of July.

Nobody had actually told me that the operation I was about to go through was similar to the one I had at Lancaster hospital; this was just a notion I had come to all on my own, again making assumptions. The operation was to remove *glands* as against the singular gland that had been taken away a couple of months earlier. But every other aspect of the operations seemed to be the same; as before I would wake up with a drain attached to the wound, and as before I would be allowed to go home once this drain had done its job. I really should learn to stop assuming things.

I came to from the operation in the recovery room with a nurse sitting beside me. She welcomed me back and guided my hand to the button that administered morphine. I can't say I was in a lot of pain, certainly nothing like the pain I was in after my hysterectomy. Of course, this could have something to do with the fact that I had learned to be nice to anaesthetists, and had not forgot to mention to him that I had no pain threshold whatsoever and that I would be really grateful if he could make sure I had as much local anaesthetic as he could fit into the wound before I was sewn up

The nurse who had been sitting by my side when I came to from the anaesthetic accompanied me back to the ward. The ward nurse asked how many times I had pressed the button for morphine.

'72 times,' she was told, and I noticed the surprised expression that passed between the two nurses.

'How many times is average?' I asked, finding that my voice was a tad slurred.

'Around 20,' the ward nurse told me.

I was in one of those beds that can be put into different positions at the press of a button, and my bed was almost in a sitting position.

'You will have to sleep sitting up for a while,' the nurse told me.

'How long for?' I asked, thinking that it would be nice to be able to lie down at some stage of the night.

'About a month,' she told me; information that I was getting for the first time. 'And we won't be letting you out of bed until tomorrow, so if you need to go just press the button and someone will bring you a bedpan.'

I recall smiling inanely at her.

'Good idea; I wouldn't let me out of bed either,' I told her, feeling like I had been on the booze. I take it that was because of my excessive use of the green button. All I needed was a karaoke machine and my evening would have been complete.

It was the following day that I found out just how long I had been in surgery. It had taken Mr Small several hours to complete the operation to remove as many glands as he could find. A drain had been inserted, as I had been told it would be, but this was no little plastic bottle, this was a bloody milk bottle!

During the night I had used a bedpan when I needed the loo, but as anyone who has ever used one of these knows, they are very uncomfortable, not to mention noisy. So I was relieved (no pun intended) that the nurse agreed for me to find my own way to the bathroom that morning, after breakfast.

The pump that had supplied me with morphine all night was removed from my hand. I was reluctant to let it go, but the nurses assured me that they would make sure I had enough pain relief throughout the day. I tucked my milk bottle into the dressing gown pocket and headed off in the direction of the communal loos.

I had already felt around the back of my head so I knew that my hair was matted with blood, even though I had thought to plait my hair prior to being taken off for surgery. But I hadn't touched the area that had been operated on, so I had no idea what it was likely to look like.

I was shocked when I came out of the toilet and looked at myself in the mirror. The T shaped wound ran horizontally from beneath my ear for about 4 inches, then down as far as my collarbone. I couldn't tell whether the wound was stitched or stapled because of the amount of blood that was caked around it. There were dozens of paper stitches (I'm sure that's not what they are officially called, but paper stitches is what we commonly know them as) along the wound and in general I looked a mess.

But of course what the untrained eye sees, and what the doctors see are two different things. When Mr Small and his team came to see me later that morning he was more than pleased with the look of the wound and I was assured that it should heal beautifully.

As hospitals go, Preston is not the worst one in the country, I'm sure of that. Not that I have stayed in all the hospitals in the country, but I would have to be blind and deaf not to hear and see the complaints that are aired about other hospitals. At Preston the food is really good, the staff are nice, and while it may not have the most up-to-date facilities I felt like I was being cared for, which is the main thing. If I were being privately treated I would always wonder if the staff were being nice to me because they were highly paid.

My first morning on the ward, I had woken feeling more hungry than I had for a long time. When the breakfast trolley came round I felt as though I could have sat in front of it and eaten until I burst. But I restrained myself and had porridge, a brown roll with butter and jam and a cup of strong coffee. The porridge in Preston hospital is wonderful, and would give any 5* hotel a run for its money, but if you want to be able to taste your coffee I recommend asking for it 'strong', otherwise you end up with a cup of 'hot'.

A while later the newspaper seller came around the ward. And I'm sure anyone who has ever had a stay in Preston hospital will agree with me that the newspaperman has got the strangest voice ever. His tone is very high pitched, his accent is from somewhere far more exotic than Preston, and coupled together these two elements combine to form a comical sound that I cannot reproduce in words so you'll just have to use your imagination.

My cousin, Kevin and his wife, Kath sent me a beautiful bunch of flowers while I was in hospital. Normally flowers are not allowed on wards anymore; this has something to do with the germs that are emitted from the water if it is not changed every seven nano seconds or so. But my flowers were in oasis and didn't need a vase so I was allowed to keep them on the window ledge next to my bed.

Later that day a young Chinese man came around the wards with a mop and stopped next to my flowers.

'What are they?' He asked me, pointing to the display. His accent was very strong, and he seemed to struggle with English as he obviously hadn't got to the word 'flower' yet.

'Flowers,' I told him, and he smiled.

'Yes, I know they are flowers,' he told me with an amused smile. 'I know these are carnations, and these are fuchsia, but I don't know what these are called' he added, gently cupping the orange flowers that I couldn't help him with the name of. I felt quite embarrassed, as I hadn't even known what the fuchsias were. His English wasn't bad after all, and his horticultural knowledge was obviously far better than mine.

I wasn't allowed to take a shower because of the wound and the drain that was inserted into it, but I had to get my hair clean somehow, so I went to the toilets and hung my head over the sink to wash the blood from my hair, changing the water over and over until it ran clear, taking care to make sure that I kept the wound area dry, which, believe me, was not easy.

Tom had asked permission to stay in the motorhome in the hospital car park, which the parking staff agreed to as we live so far away from the hospital. Great, at least I would have one visitor. Yet Tom still managed to be late for visiting!

As anyone who has ever stayed in hospital knows, camaraderie develops between patients sharing the same ward that is warm and comforting. I would hate to be in a private room while in hospital, with nobody to talk to, nobody to compare ailments/operations with. Firm friendships are made during hospital stays; patients help one another when they can, and often when they struggle to do so. Yet strangely, hospital formed friendships never seem to last for me. I don't know if it is *just* me, but, once I have gone home, I struggle to remember the names of people I share hospital wards with, unless they really stood out for some reason or another.

I'm sure that many lasting friendships are formed during hospital stays, but in the main the people we share a ward with are people whom we rarely see again.

But to me it is so important to have people around me when I am in hospital that I wouldn't dream of being in a private room

I recall one woman who was in a private room during this stay in hospital. I don't know what her operation had been, but she was carrying two milk bottle sized drains around with her whenever she left her room. But unlike me, she carried her bottles in a fancy straw bag, so that anyone who saw her would assume she was on her way to the beach. Every so often she would come out of her room and wander down the corridor, obviously in pain, and then she would walk back again, smile at anyone whose eye she caught, and then go back into solitary confinement. She seemed to want to talk to someone, but didn't know how, so instead she just went back to her room. It was quite sad really. I tried saying hello to her, but I think the wound on my neck terrified her, because she looked away quickly, muttering hello back at me before going back to her room to hide away from me. Or I could have just been a tad paranoid.

Ah well, at least she had her Patientline (now called Hospedia) TV to keep her company.

As anyone who has stayed in hospital over the past few years knows, Patientline is a system that allows patients to watch TV, play games, surf the Internet (very slowly) and make/receive telephone calls without having to leave the bed. It is outrageously expensive to use, and most people feel that they have been ripped off when they purchase a card to use the system, but everyone does it anyway because having a TV right next to your bed really helps to pass the time.

But one thing bugs me about these Patientline/Hospedia systems; it bugs me so much that I wrote to the Department of Health about it. The damn things have to be full of bugs!

Nobody bothers to clean them when new patients take over a bed.

The system consists of a TV screen on a moveable arm that is fixed to the wall over the bed. To one side of the screen is a telephone handset, and to the other side there is a remote control. When a patient is discharged from hospital the bed is stripped, and everything is disinfected... but not the TV system, because this has nothing to do with the nursing staff and it is not part of their duty to make sure that the system is germ free. I once heard a nurse say: 'thank goodness they have nothing to do with us' as she stripped a bed one day.

So when a patient leaves, they also leave whatever germs they have left on the system for the next patient to pick up when they use the remote control or the phone; or even when they adjust the position of the TV. It really doesn't take a genius to work out that germs have to be passed from patient to patient via these systems, and nobody seems to care.

The NHS is desperately trying to eradicate MRSA from hospitals in the UK... Hello!!!!

While I am a stickler for cleanliness, especially while in hospital, there are many who don't seem to give a damn. I recall being in one of the toilet cubicles one day and hearing the person in the cubicle next to me leave without washing her hands.

But it is not just people not washing their hands after using the loo that bothers me. Visitors also touch the TV systems, and bored children being entertained by the games while visiting use them. And we all know how hygienic children aren't.

But when I wrote to the Department of Health to point this out all I got by way of response was a standard letter that only told me that nobody was listening. So, whenever I go into hospital I take antibacterial wipes with me. If nobody else is going to clean the systems, then I feel I have to do it myself.

I was kept in for four days, during which time I was informed that the histology on the glands that had been removed from my neck did not show any cancerous cells; nor did the biopsies that had been taken from my tongue and from the back of my throat show any sign of cancer.

While in one way this was good news, in another way it was bad because it meant that the doctors still had no idea where the primary source of the cancer had been. Mr Small explained that sometimes the body's natural defences kill off the primary cancer, and that this could well be what had happened in my case. I took this offering and ran with it. To think that there could still be a primary source of cancer lurking somewhere was too much for the senses, it was far easier to believe that my own body had killed it off.

The drain had to come out before I could go home; otherwise I would be left with a milk bottle full of blood hanging out of my neck forever, and not all of my clothes have pockets big enough to accommodate a milk bottle. It seemed like a simple enough procedure. The drain was held in place by two stitches, which were snipped and pulled out without any pain, and then out came the tube that had been placed under my skin during the operation.

Did it hurt? Yes it bloody well did. But only for the briefest of moments, then it was gone, and I could go home. I could go home and hide where nobody would recoil in horror at the sight of my horrendous wound. But first there was a 70-mile journey to contend with.

Ten miles from home, and my bladder felt as though it was going to burst. The wilds of Cumbria are lacking in public toilets, but public houses are aplenty, even in the middle of nowhere, and so we stopped outside one such hostelry, and I went inside to ask the lady behind the bar if I could use the loo, explaining that I had just come out of hospital. It was only when I looked in the mirror in the ladies' toilet that I realised her look of terror was because the blouse that I thought would cover the wound successfully did nothing of the sort, and the bloody, stitched gash on my throat was visible, so visible that I looked like a walking experiment.

I hated the wound on my neck, and the resulting scar. The doctors may have thought it was a 'beautiful' scar, but I thought it was ugly and offensive for other people to have to look at, and so I became the queen of floaty scarves whenever I went outdoors.

I later learned that there were no stitches holding the wound together, other than the paper stitches that washed off eventually, after a couple of weeks or so. It's a good job I didn't know that it was only paper stitches holding me together; otherwise I would have been afraid to move lest the whole thing opened up again and my head fell off.

I had given up smoking again, well, almost. So long as I had a cigarette every three days or so I coped quite well the rest of the time.

Every month I had to go back to Preston to see Mr Small. Every month I had a camera shoved up my nose to make sure there was nothing worrying happening in my throat, and every month I was sent home after being told that everything looked fine, so that eventually I began to settle and accept that the operation had been a success, and that there was no cancer to be found.

I didn't always see Mr Small. Sometimes he wasn't there and I would see another doctor. One month I saw Dr Jain, a doctor I had not seen before. I sat down in front of him, steeling myself for the onslaught of the dreaded camera.

'Which nose do we usually put the camera up?' He asked me.

Who wouldn't be worried at that question? Shouldn't a doctor be aware that most people only have one nose?

2007 ended, and in came 2008, and with the New Year came a decision that it was time for me to try to get a job. I had been out of work a long time, and now that I was better it was time for me to get out into the world again instead of shutting myself in at home with my computer. My scar wasn't as noticeable, and could be easily covered up by Este Lauder's double wear foundation. My age was going to be against me. Realistically, it's not as easy to get a job at 52 as it is at 18. And I knew that I was going to have to be honest with any prospective employer with regards to my health.

Nat West offered me an interview, the job itself would be based in Barrow, but the interview was to take place in Carnforth. So off I set one morning, arriving in Carnforth in plenty of time, and with a full bladder. I'm sure my bladder has shrunk to the size of a garden pea as I have got older.

I can't say I attended this interview filled with confidence. For one thing the position came with a certain amount of responsibility, and responsibility is not something that I am particularly comfortable with. Also, I had been out of the workplace for a couple of years by this time, and I had thought I might be retired. It was only when I came through the operation that I realised I needed to get out into the world again, and that a job would be the best way of doing this.

I went into the bank and introduced myself to the girl behind the reception desk, then asked if it would be ok if I helped myself to all the money in the bank safe after donating a kidney to me.

Well, that's what anyone would have thought I had asked going by the shocked expression on her face. Her reaction did nothing to help my nerves, but I needed the loo, so what else could I do but ask? She told me to wait where I was and

went off down a corridor and through a security door. A few minutes later she

returned, having got permission from the keeper of the privy for me to piddle in their

toilets. I half expected her to ask me to sign something before showing me the way…

along the corridor, through the security door, down a stairwell, through another

security door, along another corridor at the end of which was a small office where a

solitary woman sat at a desk, working alone. I couldn't help wondering what she had

done to receive such a punishment.

The receptionist told the woman that she was taking me to the toilets; the

woman looked shocked, as though I had just pulled out a gun, and I began to think I

didn't want to work for a bank who were so bloody precious about their toilets that

they had to hide them in the bowels of the building.

Eventually the receptionist opened a door and we were there, the bank

toilets, decorated in 1970s green, complete with chipped tiles on the walls.

'Through there.' The receptionist pointed at another door, and my bladder

almost gave way there and then in relief at finally reaching our destination. I left my

bag with her, and pushed open the door.

There were two cubicles inside, and whoever had used the first one was in

dire need of medical attention and a lecture on hygiene. There is no polite way of

putting this; they had a bad case of diarrhoea and whether or not the flusher worked,

they didn't do anything to clear up the mess they had left behind.

To this day I wonder, did they think that I was responsible for making that

mess?

Luckily the other cubicle was clean; and coming out of it I looked around for

somewhere to wash my hands. The only sink was in the corner, and was a strange shape, with a single tap above it. But it was somewhere to wash my hands. However, there was nothing to dry them on, so I shook them a bit, and tapped off the excess water on my jacket.

Back in the other room the receptionist waited, and the expression on her face told me she was not waiting patiently. She gave me my handbag, with a look on her face as though I had given her a dog turd to look after, then she turned to lead me back the way we came. It was as we left the room I realised that there were two sinks just outside the door leading to the cubicles and the…

Urinal! It was a urinal! That was why it was a funny shape. It wasn't a sink at all. I had washed my hands in a urinal. And the receptionist knew what I had done.

Back upstairs I was beyond mortified. There are no words to describe my level of embarrassment that I had just washed my hands in the urinal and the receptionist either knew what I had done, or she thought that I was one of those people who didn't wash their hands after going to the loo.

Not only that, but I was also concerned that by now the entire staff of the bank was aware of the mess in the first cubicle and I was getting the blame for it. It's not like the culprit was going to own up when there was someone else to blame. Either way, the odd experience had not exactly put me in a relaxed mood for my interview. My one consolation was that she didn't have the opportunity to tell anyone else what I had done before the woman conducting my interview came out to introduce herself.

She had made it through the ranks of the bank, to a position that only a man could have held a few years ago. She was a confident woman, an intelligent woman, smartly dressed in a uniform reserved for the important members of staff. But although this well-educated, self-assured woman had progressed in her career, she had yet to discover that foundation should not end at the jaw line, and that foundation should be closely matched to the wearer's own skin tone, not to the skin tone of Lenny Henry!

I knew I was not going to get the job of counter assistant at the bank. I knew I didn't *want* the job. If the receptionist, the woman in the bowels of the building and the woman conducting the interview where examples of the staff, then I was not going to fit in.

The interview followed the same crappy, corporate line that so many interviews follow these days, and the same old questions were asked.

'Why do you want to work for Nat West?' 'Tell me about a time when you had to explain a complicated matter to someone.' 'Do you enjoy working as part of a team?'

This, and other such shite that does nothing to give the interviewer a clear picture of the applicant, was the format of the questioning.

I left the building, in the sure and certain knowledge that I had not got the job, I did not want the job, and I had just wasted half a day of my life in conversation with a woman who had yet to work out how to put on her make up.

Over the next couple of months I made a hobby out of filling in application forms. I applied for anything I thought I would be able to do, but rarely got interviews. One big problem was the town I lived in; so far away from civilisation that prospective employers seemed to doubt my ability to get to work on time.

But eventually I found a job, in customer service, contacting customers to check their eligibility for a wonderful insurance plan. Yes, in other words I became one of those really annoying people who ring you when you are in the middle of cooking tea to offer you insurance that you don't want.

Well, nobody seemed to want it from me anyway. Although I said the same words as the top sellers, reading from a carefully worded script, I was so bad at getting sales that it is something of a miracle that I wasn't sacked.

The company were really good to me, allowing me time off every month to go to my hospital appointment to have a camera shoved up my nose, to be told that everything was fine, until June 2008, when I scratched an itch on my neck and found a lump.

Head up arse again!

I went to the boss and told her what I had found, and she kindly sent me straight home to see my doctor. My GP got in touch with the hospital, and within days I was back in hospital to have lots of biopsies taken from my neck and my throat. Thankfully Mr Small decided this would be best performed under general anaesthetic. He told me I would need a week off work to recover, and my employers not only gave me the time off but also paid me for it. So I suppose I must have been making enough sales to keep them happy.

Once again I found myself in Preston hospital wearing surgical stockings and a gown, waiting for yet another operation. This time I was a little more scared; having found lumps that seemed to alarm Mr Small I was afraid that the histology would be positive this time.

But, once again nothing was found to cause any concern. It turned out that the lump was an enlarged saliva gland and that this was not unusual after the kind of operation I had the year before. So off I went back to work.

I can't say I liked my job. Sales is an area of employment that some people are born to do and others, myself included, struggle to keep performance targets at an acceptable level. It was bloody hard work sometimes. Like the time I called Mr

Umbongo (I kid you not).

'So, if I give you my bank details you will put £75,000 into my bank

account,' he said in a strong African accent when I had explained why I was ringing.

He started to give me his account number, but I had to stop him. You see, there really

are people in this world that will give their bank details to anyone who rings up and

asks for them.

A couple of months later an opening in another department within the

company became available, and I applied for it successfully. I was no longer calling

people up to offer them insurance; now the customers were calling me for advice on a

range of issues that I had been extensively trained in, and I was happy with my job at

last.

In October 2008 Mr Small was so happy with my progress that he decided I

need only attend the hospital every two months; not only that, but I could go to

Barrow hospital instead, which would mean I would just have to have a couple of

hours off work instead of a whole day. Mr Small told me I would be getting a letter in

the post to tell me when the appointment would be. I thanked him profusely for

everything he had done for me over the past year or so and went home to wait for the

letter with an appointment for December.

No letter came, and then it was Christmas, and then it was the New Year,

and then it was time to go back to work

And then I found a lump!

Then I found another lump, and another, eventually eight in a crooked row

down the side of my neck. Yet I wasn't particularly alarmed. Lumps had been found

before and they had not been cancerous, so there was no reason for me to assume these ones were. Quite the reverse, I assumed that because the lump I had found the last time was not cancerous, neither would these lumps be.

I wanted to be told that there was nothing to worry about, as I was the last time, but for that to happen I first had to get to a doctor, but this was proving to be a trial in itself.

I rang Preston hospital and was told that I should have received an appointment with Mr Mian at Barrow, but no such appointment had been given to me, not unless the letter had been lost in the post. So I rang Barrow hospital, to be told that they had not received a request for an appointment. So I called Preston again and was assured that a request had definitely been sent. So I rang Barrow again…

By this stage it was the second week in January, I had eight lumps on the side of my neck and I was becoming a little pissed off at the lack of communication from Barrow hospital.

Eventually Mr Small's secretary sorted the problem out for me and I received an appointment to see Mr Mian.

I didn't bother to take a whole day off work. The appointment was in the afternoon, so I worked until just after lunchtime and then got a taxi up to the hospital.

Like many hospitals these days, Barrow employs many Women's Institute members to help out and it was one such woman (aged approximately 104) who took my letter from me with shaking hands before telling me to take a seat.

The waiting area for the ENT department is beneath a huge, metal sculpture that hangs from the ceiling. A massive work of 'art' made from twisted metal. Did someone pay for this? Was it donated? I haven't bothered to ask, because I don't want to be told that a single penny of NHS funds was used to pay for the monstrosity that looks like a reject from a scrap-yard.

Over an hour later I was still waiting while others who arrived after me came and went. Eventually I went over to the reception desk to enquire if there was a delay and was told that there was, and was assured that my letter had been handed in to the department. So I went back to my chair, where I got talking to a woman whose appointment was almost an hour after mine.

'Who are you seeing?' She asked me, and I told her I was to see Mr Mian. 'Oh,' she said, grimacing. 'So am I?'

'What's he like?' I asked her, as if I couldn't tell by the look on her face.

'I don't like him. Last time I saw him he was so abrupt and offhand with me that I complained afterwards. I have never complained about anyone before,' she added, lest I thought her to be a serial complainer for whom nothing was good enough. 'I asked to see someone else, but I was told he was the best in his field at this hospital,' she told me.

Her words didn't fill me with confidence, but I was grateful for the heads up anyway. Then the woman who had warned me about the doctor was called in for her appointment, and I realised I had to have been overlooked, so I asked the nurse to check for me.

It turned out that the letter I handed in to reception, some 20 feet away from the waiting area for the ENT department, had been lost in transit, and if I hadn't asked I would still be sitting there now. It was at this moment that I lost confidence in Barrow hospital. Such inefficiency is unacceptable in any hospital. All they had to do was get a letter from reception to the department; then all they had to do was place this letter with the other appointment letters before calling me in. How difficult is this?

The nurse came back and apologised before asking me to come into the department where I could sit in a corridor and wait instead of sitting waiting at the waiting area. Was this an attempt at psychological trickery to make me believe that I was about to get in to see the doctor? If it was, it didn't work.

I would normally have to be poked with a sharp stick to be made angry, but this made me mad, and I sat silently fuming until I was called in to see the doctor.

What do you notice first about a person?

On this occasion the first thing I noticed about Mr Mian was his watch. It was the biggest, goldest, glitteriest watch I have ever seen in my life and I am surprised he is able to lift his right arm with the weight of it.

He examined my neck, and perhaps it is necessary to use a certain amount of pressure to determine the depth of lumps, but it hurt. He put a spatula in my mouth to look at the back of my throat, and perhaps it is necessary to exert a lot of pressure on my enormous tongue to see past it, but my tongue was pressed down so hard onto my teeth it really hurt. He made no apologies for any of this.

Then he squirted liquid up one nostril and inserted the camera to look down my throat, and credit where it is due, he performed this task without much discomfort.

'What do you think the lumps could be?' I asked him, and without batting an eyelid or changing his abrupt tone he replied:

'Cancer,' he stated flatly, showing no emotion, and my stomach went into a knot. Did he sit watching my face for a reaction? Perhaps everything went into slow motion, but it seemed as though he was studying my face for a long time. Perhaps it was only seconds.

I tried to keep my composure, but it was difficult. Usually when I go to hospital appointments Tom is with me, but this time I had told him there was no need, so I was alone as fear gripped me. Up until then, other than the gland that Miss Ahmed had removed, any lumps that had been found had been innocuous, so how could he be so certain that the new lumps were cancerous?

'What happens now?' I asked.

'I can cut them out,' Mr Mian replied, in a manner so offhand, so blasé that it was hard to believe he was talking about cancer; it was hard to believe that he was talking to a human being; it was hard to believe that he had an ounce of compassion .

'Are there any alternatives? I asked.

'You can go back to Preston if you wish,' he told me.

'I don't want to insult you by doing that,' I said, and he shrugged his indifference.

'I would not be insulted, we are all professional,' he replied. And I remember thinking that some were more professional than others. Mr Small would never have spoken to me in the manner that Mr Mian had. Mr Small would never shrug indifferently.

'In that case I will go back to Preston,' I said, relieved that I had this option.

It is not possible to reach the age I have without encountering many people in the world of medicine along the way. But I have never met any doctor with such poor people skills as Mr Mian. His attitude was disdainful and showed none of the care and compassion that I have experienced while attending Preston hospital. I felt that he really couldn't care less what I decided to do, and because of this I felt I had no option other than to choose to return to Preston, to see Mr Small, to be told that the lumps may not be cancerous, that there could be some other explanation. The lumps could be cysts, or they could be caused by scar tissue from previous operations. They could have been completely harmless.

But still, Mr Mian's words filled me with dread, and as I left his room after shaking his hand and thanking him (manners cost nothing) I felt tears well up in my eyes.

I had hardly noticed the nurse and the other lady who had been in the examination room. They had sat close by, but they were not included in any of the conversation and Mr Mian didn't need their assistance during the examination. And as he told me that the lumps were cancer, with such certainty in his voice, the world fell away and there was only he and I in the room. But as I left, the lady who had stood in the background followed me out, and as the tears started to overflow in spite of my best effort to keep them in check she put a gentle hand on my back and guided me into another room further along the corridor.

'You made the right choice,' she told me, handing me a bunch of tissues to mop up my tears. She didn't explain her words, and I doubt that she was casting any aspersions on Mr Mian's ability as a doctor; rather that she meant it was best for me to go back to the doctor who was most familiar with my case. Then again, perhaps she was only too familiar with Mr Mian's brusque manner, and considered Preston a better option for all patients.

I apologised for crying. Crying is not something that I do often and it really has to be a moving incident to make me shed tears, like weddings and funerals, or a dog being killed in a movie, even though I know it's not real. But to cry over myself... that I don't do, so I can only assume that it was Mr Mian's attitude that made me cry that day.

Isabel, as I was later to discover her name to be, gave me a hug and made sure I was ok before letting me go that day. I was also later to discover that Isabel is a specialist nurse, and that her particular speciality is cancer. But on that particular day she was simply the caring person I needed, at the right time, in the right place.

Confession time.

I got a taxi into town, went into a shop and bought 10 cigarettes and a lighter. Outside the shop I lit a cigarette and sat on a bench in Dalton Road to smoke it.

OK, at that time I was back to smoking 2 cigarettes a day; I had one in the morning before I left for work, and one in the evening when I got home. Stupid, I know. And perhaps smoking that cigarette after seeing Mr Mian that day was no worse than smoking 2 cigarettes a day. But to me it seems a particularly stupid response to being told I had cancerous lumps in my neck, even though there was no definitive proof of this as no biopsies had been taken.

As I smoked my cigarette, other people walked past smoking their own cigarettes, and I wanted to jump up and knock them out of their hands; I wanted to scream at people 'Don't you know that those things cause cancer? Are you too stupid to understand that those things kill people?' But instead I smoked my own cigarette in silence before getting up and putting the rest of the packet and the lighter into the nearest bin, feeling enormous guilt for having smoked that cigarette and mentally vowing to myself that I would never smoke another cigarette.

My appointment to see Mr Small came through quickly, and the following week I was off to Preston again. Just knowing that I was going to see Mr Small made me feel better; after all, he was the one who had allayed my fears in the past, and I was confident of his ability to do so this time.

He examined my neck from behind, and when he sat back down to write something in my notes it was impossible to deduce anything from his expression.

'I'd like to take a needle biopsy from one of the lumps,' he told me, making the considered decision that Mr Mian had failed to do before he had rashly declared the lumps to be cancerous.

I cringed at the idea, and he noticed.

'It will just be a small scratch,' he said, as he prepared the needle.

'Don't lie. I have had one of these done before,' I told him, recalling when the gentle Miss Ahmed had stuck a needle in the gland that had been removed, and how much it had hurt. But I smiled at him, and he smiled back. He had a job to do, I had to let him do his job, and so I steeled myself as he stuck the needle into my neck and withdrew a tiny bit of matter. I nearly went cross-eyed as he withdrew the needle, but then again I have no pain threshold, and other people probably wouldn't feel it nearly as much as I did.

Another appointment was made for the following week, and I decided that until I knew what the results were, I was not going to worry myself. So I continued to go to work and waited until I knew what the outcome was before panicking.

However, even when Mr Small told me that cancerous cells had been found in the biopsy he had taken and he was going to have to perform another neck dissection, I was strangely calm about the whole thing. After all, he had taken glands out before, I had survived, and I could do so again. It was beginning to feel like pregnancy; something I never wanted to go through again, but did when I had to.

During the consultation where I was given the results of the histology I was also introduced to Dr Siva.

'You may have to have some radiotherapy after the operation.' Mr Small informed me. 'Dr Siva here will be looking after you if that is the case.'

'How long will the radiotherapy last?' I asked

'Probably about three weeks.' Mr Small said. And three weeks was a time span I could deal with in my head.

My calculations went thus: three weeks to recover from surgery, three weeks of radiotherapy. All in all, I could be back at work in about six weeks, which didn't seem too bad. I shook Dr Siva's hand as I was introduced to him, and couldn't help noticing that he had a lovely smile.

To me a smile can speak reams about a person, and if Dr Siva's smile was anything to go by here we had a lovely man, caring and genuine, and with great teeth.

I can't say I lost any sleep over the news I received that day at the hospital. In fact, I slept like a top as usual. (I would love to know where that saying comes from; sleeping like a top… what kind of top? Why does it sleep?) I didn't lose my appetite and still ate well. I didn't feel sad, or worried, after all, cancer had been found in my neck before, it had been taken away, and I had been fine. So I had no reason to think otherwise this time.

No, I didn't worry at all, not until the phone call came into the office on Wednesday the 25th of February. The call was from Preston hospital, and it was to give me the date for my new operation; Friday the 27th of February, but they would like me in the day before for all the pre operation checks. This meant that I was now working my last day until I got better. This also meant that I was finally scared. Not scared of the cancer, but scared of the operation, and of the pain that was sure to follow.

That evening I went home and smoked a cigarette, the last cigarette I smoked. At the moment I doubt very much that I will ever smoke again, but only time will tell. That cigarette, like my last cigarette before my hysterectomy, did nothing to allay my fears, and served no purpose whatsoever other than to make me feel guilty for smoking it. The guilt came from letting myself down.

I don't think I am any more of a wimp than the average person when it comes to operations. I'm sure anyone would have been scared to know that their neck was going to be opened up and lumps cut out. But this had to be faced, and so I tried to do so with as much dignity as possible.

On the day of the operation all the final preparations were made as normal. A cannula was inserted into the back of my hand in readiness for the anaesthesia and any other drugs that may be necessary. Once again I walked to theatre with a nurse from the ward, with my pillow tucked under my arm. In the room outside the operating theatre, I had a word with the anaesthetist to make sure she was aware that I had no pain threshold and would need the very best pain relief she could supply. While I stood there talking to her a man came out of the operating theatre, it took a couple of seconds for me to realise that it was Mr Small. I had only ever seen him in a shirt and tie before, and he looked so different in his operating clothing.

Mr Small assured me that he would look after me, and I didn't doubt his words for a moment. I have no doubt that this man gives his all to his patients. I know he works long hours, and has to be dedicated to his job. A man with his skills could probably make a lot more money in the private sector, but no, every day he is there for his NHS patients, and he fills me with confidence in his abilities.

Surgery went on for several hours, not that I remember any of it. The next thing I knew I was in the recovery room, and then I was being wheeled back to the ward and placed on my bed by caring hands. My right hand gripped the button for the morphine pump as though it were giving life to me. And for the next few hours I drifted in and out of sleep, only slightly aware of the wound on my neck. As before, I had to sleep sitting up, but this was no hardship. I could have slept upside down, spinning round that night.

I woke up in the middle of the night in pain. As I had been asleep my finger had not been working on the button that supplied morphine to my hungry veins and the pain in my neck and shoulder demanded some sort of relief. I pressed the button, but somehow the tube that had been fitted to the end of the cannula had dislodged while I slept and I felt the precious pain relieving liquid ooze all over the back of my hand.

I needed help, so I pressed the button that summoned Nursie.

When she arrived at my bedside my brain said: 'Excuse me nurse, sorry for disturbing you in the middle of the night, but I think the morphine pump has become dislodged from my cannula.'

But my mouth said 'Uhhh!' and I pathetically tried to point at my right hand with my left. But this was really hard work, so I hoped that the nurse had the ability to pick up my telepathic transmission, as this was all I had left to beg for help with. Luckily she worked out what it was that I was desperately trying to communicate.

When I woke up again it was Saturday morning, and I knew that I was going to have to let them take the morphine pump away sometime that day, but it's amazing how attached one can become to a morphine pump under such circumstances. A nurse, who had *not* undergone several hours of surgery to *her* neck, told me that I would feel better if I had it taken off. Hah! What did she know? But eventually I had to give in and said goodbye to my good friend, the morphine pump. The nurse said that so long as I had the pump attached I would have to use bedpans. Oh, yes, I had forgotten about that rule; I let them take it away.

I deliberately didn't look in the mirror when I went to the loo that morning. I had a fair idea that this operation was a lot bigger than the last one had been, owing to the fact that I now had *two* milk bottle sized drains attached to my neck, and luckily two pockets in my dressing gown to carry them around in. I had touched the end of the scar and found that this time I was held together by staples, which induced its own kind of terror, the fear of them coming out when the wound was healed. Of course, I was also now terrified to move my neck in case the staples popped and a great, big gaping wound appeared in my neck.

I had to wash my hands after using the loo, and although I didn't want to look… I had to. And I almost reeled away from the mirror at the sight of the wound. This time it went from about an inch under my chin, along in an arc under my ear to about half way up the back of my ear; then another wound ran from this down to about an inch below my collar bone. Tiny staples held it all together, and I could have cried when I saw it, if I were the crying type, which I am not. It looked horrendous, and if I thought I looked like I was starring in Frankenstein's Bride after my last operation, hah, I had only been the understudy.

Back on the ward the breakfast trolley was on its way round, and in spite of the shock of seeing the wound on my neck, I was hungry.

Mr Small turned up just after breakfast, in yet another mode of dress I was not used to seeing him in. This time he was casually dressed in beige slacks and a striped sweater. The things a woman remembers. He was more than happy with his work and assured me that although it didn't look too tidy at that moment, the scar would be an improvement on how the last one had looked. And sometimes you just have to trust people.

I had brought a couple of books into hospital with me, including one of Jeremy Clarkson's books on how he looks at the world, but because of the drugs I was on, even this light reading was intellectually challenging.

Back home after the operation I was in a lot more pain than I had been after the last one, and there had been a bit more damage done to nerves this time. My tongue wasn't working properly; Tom, Owen and Alan were taking some amusement from getting me to say 'I did it for you Adrian.' This, apparently, is a line from a Rocky movie that I emulated rather well with my strangely shaped tongue.

I had forgotten that the right side of my face had dropped after the last operation, and this had happened again. However, unsightly as I found this, I didn't worry too much because it went back into place the last time. I was a tad concerned that the damage had been more severe this time, but I wasn't going to worry about my mouth being stuck this way, worrying unnecessarily in advance is something I consider to be a waste of time and energy.

There was a lot of pain in the shoulder area that went deeper than it did the last time. I was finding it difficult to type, and found that I could only do so for thirty-second spurts before having to rest it. It was difficult to move my right arm in any direction.

Star jumps were going to be out of the question for some time to come. Had I ever done star jumps? Yes of course I did… when I was about seven years old.

Eventually the time came for the staples to come out. This was to be done at my local doctor's surgery, by one of the local nurses. I wasn't scared about having them removed, scared doesn't even begin to describe my feelings that day. In my mind the removal of the staples would be just as painful as having staples put in, while awake. Tom came with me, and the gibbering wreck that I was laid down on the couch and turned my head to the left when the nurse asked me to. I held on to Tom's hand, squeezing for all I was worth. Why do we think it's going to help our pain to hold on tightly to something?

'That's the first one out,' the nurse said. And to be honest I hadn't felt a thing. But I continued to squeeze Tom's hand because the rest of the staples coming out were bound to put me through excruciating agony. But no, as the nurse continued to pull out the staples, with a device that looked more suited to an office desk, I didn't feel a thing. Even when it came to the last one, the one that had stuck and she had to leave to return to, I still didn't feel it coming out. I cannot tell you what a relief it was to leave the building, knowing that something I had dreaded so much was over, and that it hadn't hurt a bit. I was walking on air.

On the 24th of March, almost a month after the operation, I returned to Preston hospital for the results of the histology on the lumps taken from my neck, and to find out what was going to happen next.

I was hoping that, like the last time, nothing was going to be done, and that Mr Small would send me home, happy that he had got everything out. But this was just me being rarely optimistic. (I prefer to be a pessimist; pessimists never expect things to go right, so when things do go well, a pessimist gets a much greater buzz than the optimist, who knew things were going to go right all along.)

Cancer cells *had* been found in all of the lumps that had been removed, but I knew this was going to be the case anyway. If cancer was found in one lump it was highly unlikely that the other lumps were going to be sitting there innocently minding their own business.

Following my consultation with Mr Small we followed Dr Siva to another office so that he could explain the radiotherapy options to me. Clara, one of Dr Siva's assistants, and Andrew, the specialist cancer nurse, were also in the room and it felt less like a consultation than a meeting.

Option one: Do nothing like the last time, and keep my fingers crossed that no more lumps would appear. I call this the stupid option.

Option two: Have radiotherapy to the right side of the neck every day for three weeks. This may have killed off the primary cancer that was hiding somewhere; then again it might not if the primary source were on the left side of the neck, which could have been the case. Just because the infected glands were on the right of the neck did not necessarily mean this is where the primary source was. If I chose this option and at a later date more lymph glands became infected with cancer cells again I would not be able to repeat the radiotherapy treatment because of the risk of permanent damage to the spinal nerves. In other words, this treatment might kill off the primary cancer; it might not. This option is the gambler's choice, and I have never been much of a gambler.

Option three: Six weeks of intensive radiotherapy to both sides of the neck, with one day of chemotherapy each week. I was told that this option would cause extreme pain and that I would need to have a feeding tube fitted to my stomach because it was doubtful that I would be able to eat near the end of the treatment.

Dr Siva didn't pull any punches as to the extreme pain I would go through with this treatment. He explained that I would have to take morphine as the pain worsened, but he assured me that throughout it all I would be closely monitored and would be given all the pain relief I needed in order to cope with the pain.

There would be other side effects of the treatment that Dr Siva warned that I might find difficult to cope with. For instance, he told me that I would lose my taste buds, and that while they would come back eventually, it may take up to a year for them to return fully.

A dry mouth would also be a side effect I would have to learn to cope with, as this was likely to be a permanent consequence of the treatment. It was to be much later that I was to realise that a dry mouth also meant that eating would be out of the question.

I asked Dr Siva if I would be able to speak after the treatment, bearing in mind he had told me that my mouth would be permanently dry, and he assured me that I would, that I would be able to use fake saliva. The idea of fake saliva makes people cringe, until I point out that it is only chemicals; that there is not a production line somewhere, made up of people spitting into bottles!

I was also told that the treatment would burn the skin on my neck, like sunburn only worse. This skin on my neck would be likely to crack and bleed eventually, but again, they would give me some cream to deal with it and in my head so long as I used this cream my neck would be fine. I was choosing to be optimist over pessimist at this stage.

I may have been given three options, but realistically there was only one and that was option three. I couldn't take chances with my life by taking option two, and if I took option one and did nothing… well, eventually I was going to have to face option two and three again, probably following even more surgery, so the obvious choice was to get the worst treatment out of the way.

But I was scared, really scared, more scared than I could admit to anyone but myself. Yet still I did not cry, not even when I was alone. The only time I cried throughout the whole ordeal was the day I met with Mr Mian. I was tired too; owing to the fact that it was very difficult to sleep because of the pain in my shoulder. It seemed that no matter what way I lay, eventually my shoulder stiffened. It felt as though I had been busting doors in with my right shoulder.

I needed some sort of help with my fear, and so I went in search of the Macmillan website, but I found this to be extremely depressing. I appreciate that the forum in this site is probably a great source of comfort to many people, but I wasn't planning on dying. I just wanted some advice on how to cope with what I was about to go through.

I trawled through the list of members of the site, desperately trying to find someone with the same problem as myself. I needed to ask someone how it all was, how did they cope, did they have any magical tips to give me that would help me through? And this is how I found Jane.

Jane is, in my opinion, a lovely person who will definitely get her wings when she goes to Heaven. Jane did not go through head and neck cancer herself, but her husband David had exactly the same problem as me, complete with an occult primary source, a year earlier. I wrote to her through the messaging service on the website and she responded almost immediately.

Although Jane works, is a mother of two and is a busy lady she offered to help me in any way she could throughout my treatment. She said she would be there for me along the way, and to date she has proven to be an important part of my support structure. Whenever I have been worried or scared, I have written to Jane and she has got straight back to me with advice based on David's experience. It gave me hope that David had not only come through his ordeal but is back at work and living a normal life. To date I have not met Jane, and I don't know if I ever will. I don't know if Jane will turn into a lifelong friend or if she is someone who has come into my life to help me through this one period. Whichever, I am so grateful for Jane's support and will never be able to repay her for her kindness.

I also went looking for a book to help me through. But there wasn't one. I found lots of books by celebrities, or by doctors, and one or two by people with dubious mental abilities, but nothing by someone who had been down the NHS road to recovery. I wanted a book by someone ordinary, someone like me, but it seemed that no such book existed, and so I decided to write my own. If nothing else it would keep me occupied throughout my treatment.

I was scared, bewildered, and didn't know my arse from my elbow. Yes, Jane was prepared to help in any way she could; yes, I had family and friends who would be there for me whenever I needed them; but still I felt alone. I felt like a small child who needed to be told: 'There there, it will be alright.' But I was a growed-up (sic), not a child, and I had to deal with this somehow.

My way of dealing with this was going to be to write about my experiences, in the form of a diary, recording what happened and when, and if this diary can help someone else through this treatment in the future, then so much the better.

Chapter three – The Treatment

Damn, damn, damn. These were the words on my mind as I woke up this morning at just gone 7.30 while the rest of the world was having a well-deserved Sunday lie-in. I didn't want to be awake; I wanted to be fast asleep and dreaming nonsense. I wanted to be far away from the reality that wakefulness brings to me every morning as soon as I open my eyes. Not for me the luxury of snuggling under the duvet for another hour of Zzzs. No, this shite is filling my thoughts, every waking moment of every bloody day!

People keep telling me 'You'll come through this.' 'What doesn't kill us makes us stronger.' 'You're so brave.' … and other such platitudes because they really don't know what else to say. I have no doubt that what they really think is 'Oh my God, you poor thing, it must be really terrifying for you.' But because my friends and family care about me, they revert to clichés. Bless them, what else is there to do?

But in my head it's a different matter; there is no bravery in my head. In my head there is fear, there is dread, there is a desire to get on a plane and fly as far away as possible… there is a need for all of this to be over. Yet, at the moment, it feels as though the future is a distant destination.

I don't know what to do with my days now that I am not going to work. I know I can't go back because I am going to be up and down to Preston hospital as and when they send for me. Also, it is not possible for me to type for long periods of time, certainly not for eight hours a day. Physically it is not possible for me to go to work, but mentally I wish I were there.

I would take Molly dog for walks to pass the time, but as she likes to try to protect me from marauding Yorkshire terriers and border collies… it can get rather hair-raising. Molly is a beautiful Staffi who has no idea of her own strength. Anyone but me can take her for a walk without any problems. When anyone else takes her for a walk she plays with other dogs; when I take her for a walk she wants to kill other dogs, so passing the time walking Molly is not really an option.

Tuesday 7th April 2009

I had another visit to the hospital today. Two appointments had been sent out to me; one with a Mr Barber, an oral surgeon, and another with a nurse who is going to explain how the feeding tube is going to be fitted. It took me some time to work out that 'oral surgeon' is a fancy name for a well-qualified dentist. Actually, to be honest, I didn't work it out until I walked into the consulting room and realised that this was a dentist's surgery.

I have a morbid fear of dentists. The only one I trust is Joan Stephenson; the only dentist I have ever come across who accepts without question my need to be sedated during any procedure, even cleaning my teeth. I don't mean that I need to be sedated every day when I clean my teeth, only when they are being scraped in that torturous way that dentists do. When I have to go to see Joan she has a tray ready with a syringe full of magic liquid that sends me off to sleep so that she can perform whatever heinous task necessary.

My dread of dentists came about because of a woman in Workington. I wish I could remember her name because I would gladly reveal it here, but I seem to have blanked it out in my mind as one does with the finer details of trauma. I was having two teeth out on the day in question, but the anaesthetic hadn't worked on one of them. I realised this as soon as she started to remove it, and no doubt she realised to too by my reaction, but she just kept pulling anyway. The pain was agonising, and to this day I want to go back and punch her.

After pulling out my tooth with no pain relief she sent me off home. My husband was at a local scrap-yard while I was having my teeth out, and I was to ring him on his mobile phone when I needed to be collected, but when I asked at reception if there was a phone I could use, I was directed to a phone booth some streets away. But I was in pain, I was in shock, I was in a strange town, and I couldn't find the phone booth.

There was a pub on a corner, and I wandered in thinking that they may have a public telephone I could use. There were no customers inside, just the landlady who was behind the bar. She looked up, and then came out from behind the bar to guide me over to a chair. This lady sold booze for a living, but unlike the butcher of Workington she could see that I was in some distress. She called my husband for me, and made me wait where I was. I have no idea what this lady's name was, but her compassion moved me that day.

Anyway, that's how I ended up being terrified of dentists, as I explained to Mr Barber. But he was understanding, and kind. He explained to me that when I have the radiotherapy treatment that the blood supply to my jaw will be reduced, and that if I were to need to have any teeth out at a later date there could be a possibility that the socket may not heal properly afterwards. Worse than that, there may also be the possibility that the wound could become infected and that surgery may be the only way to remove any infection. This is why any teeth that show signs of damage or deterioration should be removed prior to radiotherapy taking place.

I was not remotely confident that Mr Barber was going to find my few remaining teeth in good condition. Although I took care of the teeth that were left, I had been made aware of the fact that I suffered from gum disease while I was only in my twenties, and as I had most of them replaced by plastic ones because of numerous abscesses over the years, I knew there was every chance that the x-ray was going to highlight some problems in that area. And I was right; two back teeth needed to be removed, to avoid further complications in the future.

'We can do it under sedation this afternoon, or you can come back on Friday,' Mr Barber told me. And while all I really wanted to do was to run in the direction of the exit, and to keep running like Forest Gump, I heard myself saying that I would have it done that afternoon, the prospect of waiting until Friday filled with dread of the procedure was an even worse option than facing up to it there and then. Besides, they were agreeing to sedate me, so at least I wouldn't know anything about it.

Hah! I don't know what kind of happy juice they use at Preston hospital, but it's not as good as Joan Stephenson's. The effect of the sedation was like drinking a few glasses of Lambrini, whereas Joan's happy juice is more like a good bottle of scotch. When Joan sedates me I don't remember a thing afterwards, but from the procedure at Preston I can recall the needles going into my gums, and that horrible feeling of the teeth coming out; the pressure followed by a popping feeling. Ok, enough said about that, just the memory of it is giving me the heebie-jeebies.

My next appointment was with one of the nurses from the endoscope department who was going to explain the finer details of having the PEG feeding tube fitted. I had looked this up online and had found a story about a ten-year-old boy who had problems eating and so had to have one of these tubes fitted. Ok, so I know that the story was written in a way that would help children through the same procedure, but as I said earlier, that's what I felt like at the time, a small child in need of childlike comfort. So when I read this story I decided that if this little boy could do it, then so could I.

They don't sugar things up at Preston hospital. And while there are some things I would rather not know, I appreciate that when it comes to things like having a feeding tube fitted, it's better to know in advance than to have things sprung on me at a later date.

Dr Siva had already made it clear that the radiotherapy is likely to make my throat so sore and swollen that I may not be able to eat or drink. In which case I will have to be fed via a tube in my stomach. (*Apparently it's not ok to shove chocolate éclairs and Big Macs down this.*) Once again I had assumed the process, and in my head it was done under general anaesthetic.

Wrong! Because the tube is inserted through the mouth and down the gullet into the stomach before being pushed through a slit they make in the tummy, I will only be sedated for the procedure. Nursie explained to me that I would need to swallow the endoscope, which she described as about the size of a large marble, and that as it is shoved down my throat I could feel as though I am choking. Only for a couple of seconds, but still this is yet another prospect that fills me with dread. The nurse told me that I will not remember anything of the procedure afterwards, but that doesn't help my fear now… yet another terror that I know I have to face… not bravely, but with a feeling of dread.

Thursday 9th April 2009

An easy day today; or so I thought when I was called at home and asked to attend the hospital for a CT scan. I was told to report to the radiotherapy department, but still I didn't cop on to the fact that this was unusual. I have had plenty of CT scans in the past, and they are relatively quick, and completely painless, so I didn't see there was anything to worry about.

I rang the surgery the day before to book transport, owing to the fact that the gear box is threatening to drop out of my car at any moment. And I know that when it does go it will not be outside a garage, or even near a lay-by. No, when the gearbox finally comes to a grinding, crashing end it will be on a blind bend on a country road, or in fast flowing traffic on the motorway. The God of 'Oh Really' will see to that one. And then, as I am not a member of any breakdown service, it will cost an arm and a leg to get it to the nearest garage, which will be so far from where the car breaks down that I will need an extra mortgage just to pay the tow-in fee. No, far safer to get transport provided by the NHS. Besides, it is free and in my car it costs around £30 per journey.

There was another cancer patient in the car when it arrived, a neighbour of a cousin of mine who was having radiotherapy after going through a mastectomy and chemotherapy... I'll call her Mary. Mary is a nice, chatty woman, and even though she has lost a breast and all of her hair she remains upbeat. She tried to give me tips on coping with the loss of taste, recommending tomato soup as something she could taste even when she couldn't taste anything else.

If only she could have given me some tips on coping with the fear. For at the moment it the worst part for me. I don't know if it's normal to feel gut wrenching, throat tightening fear at the prospect of full on radiotherapy for occult (hidden) head and neck cancer, but I do know that it is filling my head to the extent that I am seriously considering asking my doctor for Valium or something. There has to be some sort of drug that can stop me from being so utterly terrified.

At the radiotherapy department I was given a form to fill in; asking me for the same information I had already given dozens of times, name, address, religion etc., and was given a card that entitled me to a free hot drink whenever I have to attend the department. I never know what to put on these forms where they ask what religion I am. Do I put 'lapsed Catholic'? There is never enough room for me to explain how I feel about religion, so I always leave it blank.

I'm not against religion; each to his/her own, but I only go to church when I have to and I only pray when I'm feeling desperate. Like that song by The Script '... praying to a God that I don't believe in...' While I would love to believe that there is a God out there, listening to me, watching over me, and helping me in times of need, I find it very difficult to believe that such a God would allow the suffering and pain that goes on in the world that He is supposed to have created. The concept of a God creating a beautiful world and then allowing it to be tainted by evil is not something I can get my head around. The notion of a compassionate God allowing children to suffer is not something I can comprehend.

I do believe that Jesus was real, and that he walked this Earth for a reason. I do believe that what he said made sense, and that he tried his best to make others understand that if only we could be decent to one another that the world would be a much better place. In its simplest form, the teachings of Jesus are right and good. But sadly religion enters into the equation, believers start to argue over which God is real, and somehow the teachings of Jesus get pushed aside in the name of self-righteousness.

When I am faced with a moral dilemma I often ask myself: What would Jesus do? And very often the answer helps me out.

Perhaps Jesus is still out there somewhere, watching, and shaking his head in disbelief at the evil men (and women) do to one another. Perhaps he does answer the prayers of the faithful and helps to bear suffering. But my mind cannot get to grips with the idea of Jesus helping *everyone* who prays to him; after all, this is hardly going to be an orderly queue. So if Jesus does help those in need of him, those who ask for his help, perhaps it is a first come first served basis. In which case, I'm sure there are people out there in greater need than me.

I envy those who believe in, and trust in God. It must be wonderful to have this strength to rely on in times of need. But belief is not something that can be forced. Belief in God is love of God, and love is not something that anyone can simply decide to have.

So, when it comes to filling out the little box that asks for religion… there isn't the space, so I leave it blank. Then I worry, because if there is a God out there, and if at some stage of my life I need the last rites performed on me, will anyone bother to send for a Priest? Ah, such dichotomy. But at the moment I think I have other things to worry about.

When I arrived at the radiotherapy department the receptionist told me where to go to wait for my appointment and I followed her directions to a little seating area where signs on the walls said 'quiet area'. But either the woman sitting next to me had not seen the signs or she really thought that by talking incessantly to her husband in what she thought were hushed tones was being 'quiet'. If that was being quiet then it was only in her world. Or perhaps I was feeling just a little tetchy. No, let's blame the woman who was chattering away about her neighbour's garden, the milkman's inability to get the delivery to her house in time for breakfast, the jumper she was knitting for her daughter… I felt like screaming at her: 'For fuck's sake, buy your milk from the supermarket!' and 'Have you not noticed the notice that was put on the wall for you to notice?' But I didn't, I just waited quietly because perhaps talking constantly was just her way of dealing with the stress of it all.

She finally went quiet when her husband was called into the radiotherapy room just beside the seating area, and she sat flicking through a magazine until he came out again, happily announcing that it had been his final treatment. I noticed he had a red patch across the top of his forehead and wondered if he had a brain tumour, if that was what they were treating. If so, who could blame his wife for being nervous that she had to chatter constantly? I chided myself for being so impatient with the woman who was probably just dealing with things in her way.

This was my first visit to the radiotherapy department, and try as I might, I couldn't help thinking that everyone around me, apart from the staff, had cancer, and it was a horribly depressing thought. I really did not want to be there at all, no matter how nice they tried to make it, for me the area had a feel of doom and gloom to it that no amount of nice decoration was going to overcome. Perhaps over time I will feel differently; perhaps as I visit the department on a daily basis it will come to feel familiar; perhaps I may even get around to reading some of the many 'thank you' cards that are pinned to the wall. Surely these have to be an optimistic indication of how many people are saved by this treatment.

They seem to be on top of the appointment schedule at the radiotherapy department; which is good because it is stressful enough having to go there for treatment without having to sit around waiting for hours. Not that I have ever minded waiting to see a doctor at the hospital. I know they don't leave me sitting there on purpose, so I am a very patient patient.

'Lynn Connolly.' I looked up from the year old copy of Mojo magazine, and the interview with Nick Cave that I wasn't really all that interested in (Although I do like Nick Cave and the Bad Seeds, particularly songs like Red Right Hand and Opium Tea, but it's difficult to concentrate on trivia when your mind wants to focus on the fear at hand.), to see the young radiotherapist smiling across at me. I smiled back; telling myself that there was nothing to worry about, I was only there for a CT scan, and even if they wanted to inject me with dye, I knew what to expect, and it wasn't the most traumatic treatment I had ever been through. After having my throat cut open, laying down on a table and going through a hole was a piece of cake.

'Could you take everything off to the waist please?' She said as we went inside.

'*What, in front of him?*' I said in my mind, noticing the male radiologist over by the scanner machine. But I didn't voice my thoughts; after all I'm sure he was not exactly frothing at the mouth at the idea of seeing a middle-aged woman's boobies. I told myself that I am lucky my boobs are not on level with my belly button as they are with many women my age; then I told myself that this was hardly a situation where the fullness of breasts mattered; it was not a shoot for a page 3 picture. I turned my back on the man to try to keep a bit of privacy for as long as possible, only to find that I was facing a mirror.

Who the hell decided that a mirror was necessary there? After all, I was highly unlikely to want to do my make up and keep the radiologists waiting. The female radiologist handed me a sheet of paper towel to cover my embarrassment with.

I had expected this scan to follow the same format as the other ones: get undressed in a cubicle, put on a gown, have scan done. But here there was no cubicle, and the nearest thing to a gown I was offered was the piece of paper towel to put over my boobs. Not that this made any real difference because they kept lifting this up to make sure that the laser was pointing at the correct area, whatever the correct area was. No, I just had to grit my teeth, tell myself that they saw boobs of all shapes and sizes, all day every day, and that my boobs didn't matter a jot to them; it was only I who was dying off from the embarrassment.

Next came yet another lesson in why it is not a great idea to get every bit of information I need from the Internet. I had already been told that I would be having a mask made to protect my face during the treatment. I had looked this up on t'Internet and had seen pictures of how the mould is made for the mask. So when I was informed that this is what I was there for I didn't mind too much.

This technique uses a special kind of plastic. The plastic is heated in warm water so that it becomes soft and pliable. It is put onto your face so that the plastic gently moulds to fit your face exactly. It feels a little like having a warm flannel put onto your face. You can still breathe easily, as the plastic will not cover your nose or mouth. Once the mesh has moulded and become hard (which takes a few minutes) the mask is taken off. It is then ready to be used when you have your treatment.

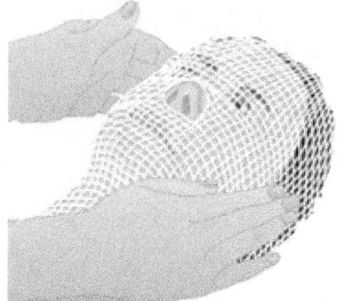

A warm plastic mesh is put onto your face so that the plastic gently moulds to fit your face

That doesn't look too bad does it? Going by the picture it is obviously a piece of light mesh, and as I was informed by this article that it was a bit like having a warm flannel placed on my face, so I wasn't unduly concerned about the process.

For me, and I am sure many other people, being informed of what is going to happen, being able to prepare for any treatment that may be carried out, is very important. Generally I have found that being in possession of the full facts often means that the actual treatment or procedure is not as bad as I anticipated. So it is my own fault that I was not fully informed about the mask; I could have asked for more information in more detail instead of relying on t'Internet. Then again, someone could have told me!

Having the hot, (not warm) heavy sheet of plastic dumped on my face was rather traumatic. It was like having a great big, hot, wet fish dumped on my face. (Not that I have ever had a hot, wet fish dumped on my face.) It was nothing like the gentle experience described in the article I found on the Internet. The lump of hot, heavy plastic was then moulded to my face and neck, quickly before it got cold.

Maybe my imagination ran away with me, as it so often does, but I recall thinking about people who say they have been abducted by aliens and experimented on.

Perhaps the oncologists don't see the making of the mask as a particularly traumatic experience compared to everything else the cancer patient has to go through, but for me it was a shock to the system that would have been far less harrowing if I had been told exactly what it would be like, and perhaps shown an example of the material used to make the mould before the day in question. I wonder if this is the difference between private and NHS patients; are the private patients given more information?

'I'm just going to tattoo a little dot on your chest,' the female radiologist told me. 'Is that ok?' She asked, and then explained that it was so that the machine could be lined up properly when my treatment was taking place. I could hardly refuse.

'Just a little scratch,' she said.

I am sure that if a doctor or a nurse were about to stab me with a six-foot spear they would still say 'Just a little scratch.' And nine times out of ten they are not being entirely truthful. As many times before, and since, the 'little scratch' felt like a sharp cut with a razor blade, but the pain was only for a second.

When the scan was over I was given a sheet of paper with a list of the treatments I am going to have. The first dose of radiotherapy is due to b e given to me on Wednesday the 22nd April, the day after I get back from my curtailed trip to Dublin. Then there will be one treatment, lasting only a few minutes, 5 days a week, with the last treatment being on 4th June. I will have every weekend off. I will have to make my own transport arrangements for any Bank holidays as apparently the transport system doesn't work on these days unless it is for dialysis patients. It is important to provide transport for radiotherapy patients unless it is a national holiday. Am I the only one seeing something odd in this?

My next visit to Preston is due on 17th April, for verification of the mask. I take it that means to make sure that the mask fits properly. Until then… all I can do is wait.

Thursday 16th April.

I woke up this morning (words that ring like the start of a bad blues song in my head; there was a time that I would have written a song about all of this) and the same dread slapped me in the face as it has each morning since the day that I made my decision to go ahead with this treatment. It's a horrible, sick feeling in the pit of my stomach, a fear that will not go away, no matter what distractions I employ.

And yet I still have a sense of humour. Strange that. I can watch reruns of Friends on TV, and even though I know what is going to happen I still laugh. I still get jokes, I still see the funny side of things, but at the same time I am filled with fear of what is going to happen. My life is a living oxymoron.

I tell myself that the effects of the treatment are transitory, that in a very short period of time it will all be over, but it doesn't help. Nor does it help when I get messed around by the people I am trusting to make me well. Not that I feel ill in any way.

Yesterday I had a phone call to tell me that the radiotherapy treatment is now going to start on the 27th of April instead of the 22nd. However, this doesn't give me any time off, as I still have to report to Preston on the 22nd to have the feeding tube fitted the following day. The procedure itself will take place on the 23rd and I will stay in hospital until Saturday the 25th. Then I will have Sunday at home before going back to Preston on the 27th to start the radiotherapy. I assume this will also put my finish date back another few days, and I sigh at the prospect.

Right now I should be looking forward to my trip to Dublin, delighting in the anticipation of the Pink concert and in finally meeting Lee Dunne face to face. But all of this is overshadowed by the fear.

I just checked out the word 'fear' in the thesaurus, I so hate using the same word over and over, but then I thought 'What the heck, fear is what it is, so why bother trying to dress it up as anything other?'

Perhaps one day I will look back on what I have written here and smile at how scared I was over something that I managed to get over quite well. Perhaps I will look back and feel thoroughly justified in being so scared. It remains to be seen.

For now I can only write of what I experience and how I am feeling as and when it happens. There is little point in my coming to this every day and saying how scared I am; I think I have managed to convey that already.

My shoulder is gradually feeling better. When I say 'better' I don't mean that it is pain free, just that it is not a constant excruciating paint as it was just after the operation. I still can't lift anything remotely heavy with my right arm, chores like ironing cause lots of extra pain and the scar is still very visible, but the pain is not as bad when I am (I almost said 'relaxed', but I am not relaxed at all) not doing things, so that's something at least.

One aspect of recovering from surgery that I am finding difficult to deal with is the boredom. I have Charles Dickens to thank for that. Apparently, according to my cousin Suzanne, it was Dickens who first used this word in the context of being tired of something, in the novel Hard Times. Were it not for Dickens I would simply be looking for things with which to fill up my time. Instead, I am whinging about being bored.

Most mornings I will try to write something here. Some days I just look at the screen and close it all down again. The Internet is a good distraction. I play Literari In Yahoo games, it's like Scrabble, but altered so that there is no infringement of trademark or copywrite laws.

In the afternoons I find myself drawn, in a macabre way that resembles rubbernecking on the motorway after a crash, to Jeremy Kyle's show on TV. Not that I like it, but it is… entertaining is the wrong word to use in just the same way that entertaining would be the wrong word to use to describe rubbernecking after a motorway crash. As the Jeremy Kyle show is a part of my world at the moment, it seems relevant to voice my opinion of it here.

For those of you who have never seen the Jeremy Kyle show; Jeremy Kyle is judge and jury to people who apply to go on his show for DNA tests to prove who the father of children are, or for lie detector tests to prove or disprove partners' and relatives' deceptions. It's like the Gerry Springer show of England. A judge once called the show 'human bear baiting' yet still Jeremy Kyle stands on the stage and announces 'This is *my* show.' with not only pride in his voice but also with an unnerving touch of what comes across to me as megalomania.

Jeremy berates his 'guests' over their lifestyles, their sleeping around, their gambling addictions, drug and drink addictions, their lies and their laziness. He orders people off set saying things like 'Get off my stage, you disgust me.' with a frown on his forehead that a Klingon from Star Trek would be proud of.

However, Jeremy does not come across to me as the brightest bulb in the economy pack. He regularly says things like '…you are here for a lie detector.' missing out the word 'test' on the end of the sentence, so that I get a mental image of the track suited, toothless guest leaving with a lie detector machine under his arm at the end of the show. '… you are here for DNA.' is another sentence that would benefit from the word 'test' being tacked onto the end. Unless that is, the guests really *do* get sent home with some DNA; who knows what happens backstage?

Kyle is regularly slated by the media; labelling him 'The Ringmaster' of what could rightly be described as a circus. The guests on the show are, more often than not, dysfunctional people who need help to sort out their lives. Some argue that the people who appear on the Kyle show know what they are letting themselves in for, that the show's format is already well known. But I have to ask how desperate these people have to be in their quest for a solution to their problems to allow themselves to be humiliated by Kyle for the sake of his own ego and TV ratings.

Jeremy Kyle is all part of my treatment and healing process. The more I watch of his show the more I want to get back to work.

A couple of days in Dublin.

This holiday was planned months ago, long before I found further lumps in my neck that necessitated surgery and radiation therapy. When it was announced on RTE that Pink would be playing at the O2 on the night of 19th April it seemed like a wonderful way to spend my birthday. But sadly the tickets were all gone when I tried to book. But as the demand for tickets had been so great another concert was announced for the 20th and I managed to get three tickets for my daughter Melissa, my Granddaughter Jade and me. The plan was to go to Dublin for a week, and have a good break, but as it turned out we had to cut it down to 2 and a half days because of having to get back in time for my feeding tube to be fitted before the radiotherapy was to start. I might not be able to put my worries to the back of my mind completely, but I was certainly going to try.

We arrived at Manchester airport for 9.00 am on the Sunday morning, the day of my 53rd birthday and did what all budding party animals do at such times, we headed straight for the bar after checking in our cases. I ordered a bottle of white wine.

'Would you like a bucket?' The barman asked.

'No, a bottle will do fine,' I replied with a smile, even though I knew he meant would I like a bucket of ice to put the bottle into. Realistically it wasn't going to last long enough to get warm, but we graciously accepted the offer of an ice bucket and settled down into some leather seats in order to watch people go by.

I love people watching, I have done ever since I was a small girl, when I would sit on the wall outside our house and watch people go by, wondering about their lives, who they were, where they came from, where they were going... there is so much we do not know about people who pass us in the street or at the airport.

When I was younger, and of an age when I still went out to pubs at night, a friend and I used to play a game whereby when people came into the pub we would guess what they did for a living. And sometimes, if enough alcohol were consumed by the end of the night, we would go up to these strangers and ask them if we were right, and invariably we were way off the mark. It was a lesson in never judging people by what they looked like, because the clothes people wear can never reveal the person inside, nor can how they style their hair tell anything about the person. Although, in the case of the guy in the pilot's uniform, we may have been pretty much close to the mark.

The screens announced that our plane was boarding so we finished up our drinks and made our way to the security area.

'Sorry, you can't take that book on board,' a security man told Jade, and she looked at the book in her hand with a look of despair that she may have to abandon Pete Doherty's autobiography. The security man smiled, it was only his way of alleviating the boredom of his job. Although, personally speaking, I think Pete Doherty, and his book, should be banned from everywhere!

Jade went through the security barrier, and set off the alarms. A female security officer started to frisk search her, and Melissa hurried through the barriers herself to be with her daughter, and she also set off the alarms and had to be frisk searched.

In no time at all we were on the plane, and less than half an hour later we were fastening our seatbelts for landing. During the flight a flight attendant came around with magazines that most people declined, not I. At the prices they charge to put four ounces of luggage on board I was taking any freebies that went with the deal. And then I was home. I sigh when I type that because for me the feeling of landing in Dublin, either at the airport or at the docks is one that I cannot describe to anyone who has not lived away from the place they call home. Arriving in Dublin gives me a sense of belonging that I cannot feel anywhere else in the world. I have lived in this town where I am now for 26 years, but still it is Dublin that I yearn for. In Dublin I am surrounded by people with the same accent as me, people who will not recoil in horror if I say 'fuck', people with a sense of humour that I don't believe can be found anywhere else in the world. Dublin is unique; it is a bustling city, yet people still have time for you, there are places where you can stroll at your leisure, and you can wear what you want… there will always be someone wearing something far more out there.

A taxi into town, a quick wash and brush up, and it was time to see what shops were open. Dublin is shopping heaven, no matter what your budget you will find yourself travelling home with far more than you arrived with. There are the trendy shops, the designer outlets and my favourite, Penny's. I love Penny's, Primark's head office, and I usually come back from Dublin with heaps of clothing from there. Not this time though, this time I had to restrict myself because I have been told that I am probably going to lose weight with the treatment, and as I don't know exactly how much weight I am going to lose I had to restrict my spending on this trip. That didn't stop Melissa and Jade from carrying armfuls of goodies to the checkout though.

We walked down O'Connell Street in the sunshine, just soaking up the city, and made our way to The Arndale to book for dinner that evening. OK, we know that The Arndale is tourist heaven, but we get sucked in there on every visit to Dublin just the same. They play Irish music, and later on Irish dancers entertain the audience. The food is not the best in town, but it's edible and filling. Then it was back to the hotel for a little rest before getting ready for our night out to celebrate my birthday.

Arriving back at the Arndale we were shown across the floor of the main bar and through a set of double doors by a member of staff. We felt as though we were being ushered back out again. Normally we had our meal in the main room, where the entertainment took place, but apparently things had changed since our last visit and now, when anyone books for dinner, they are shown to a restaurant downstairs.

We followed where the member of staff pointed, down a gloomy set of wooden stairs, as the smell of fish got stronger, and stronger. I have always hated the smell of fish. I used to avoid Moore Street like the plague on a Friday morning, but as we went deeper into the bowels of the Arlington it felt as though I were right back there, in the 1970s, with the women calling out the price of the fresh cod and plaice as I hurried past, gagging. The closest I get to serving fish in my house is fish fingers.

Downstairs we found a deserted restaurant, in almost total darkness but for the rows of tea light candles that lined the tables. The only people in the darkened room were the waiters, all of whom seemed to be Indian, and the smell of fish was completely overpowering. It was like walking into a rather surreal Indian restaurant where somebody had decided that curry was off the menu. We were met by a Maitre'd who offered to show us to a table. Melissa looked at me in horror; horror that I am sure was reflected right back at her.

'I'm sorry,' Melissa said in her normal forthright manner. 'I can't stay down here, it stinks of fish.' And I'm so glad she had the nerve to say it because it gave me the courage to agree.

'Me neither, I really can't stand the smell of fish,' I agreed with my daughter in a tone I tried to make sound apologetic. The Maitre'd looked somewhat taken aback.

'If you like there is a carvery upstairs, you could eat there,' he offered, not sounding insulted by what we had said.

We thanked him, and assured him it was nothing personal. Which, looking back now, was a rather strange thing to say, and seemed to insinuate that the smell of fish was emanating from him.

Back upstairs we found a table, ordered drinks, and made our way over to the carvery where there was not a piece of fish in sight. It was self-service, but we didn't mind carrying our own food to our table. It was a tad dry, and I couldn't finish mine, but I didn't care, I was in Dublin, I was at the Arlington (where I knew there would be ample entertainment to make up for the dry food), it was my birthday, and I was with my girls. Ok, I could have asked for more, I could have asked for more of my family to be there, but as that was not possible, I revelled in the company, the ambiance and the entertainment. And I think I was rather successful at putting my forthcoming troubles to the back of my mind.

I think I may have drunk a little more wine than I had intended to. I had a great night, we sang along to the songs, the band played The Ballad of James Connolly for me, and I happily clapped along as the dancers took to the stage. But the journey from the Arlington back to the hotel is just a little vague in my head. I can remember talking to a Norwegian couple outside the Arlington, and to a girl called Carol who we met inside. Carol had been to Pink's first night at the O2 and had wanted to carry on partying afterwards but her friends all went home and abandoned her in town. So she had found her own way to the Arlington, had met Melissa outside when she had gone out for a cigarette, and had joined us at our table. She was a hoot, a proper bundle of fun, and I gave her my email address at the end of the night. Sadly she didn't get in touch as yet, but she was memorable nonetheless.

Allegedly, I sang, or tried to sing, all the way back to the hotel, but I couldn't remember the words of songs so I had to keep starting new ones. But I only have Melissa and Jade's word for this. I woke up at about 5 am, and as ever when I am in Dublin, I couldn't get back of to sleep and only dozed until about 7 when I decided I might as well get up.

In spite of the heavy night before, we all made the most of the buffet breakfast, knowing that we needed sustenance to carry us through a morning of shopping before meeting Lee Dunne for lunch later on.

Lee had left a message with the desk at the hotel and I had rung him to arrange where we would be meeting; and I couldn't wait. We had been writing to one another quite regularly for nearly two years. I had sent him a copy of my book, signed of course, and he had sent me a signed copy of The Barleycorn Blues.

Our arrangement to meet for lunch would be our first opportunity of meeting in person, and I was excited at the prospect. I had been a Lee Dunne fan many years before, and had read lots of his books; Goodbye to the Hill, Does your Mother etc., and I was more than a little star-struck at the idea of meeting up with him, not as a fan but as a friend.

Several shoe shops and clothes shops later, Melissa and Jade found the outfits they needed for the Pink concert, and some Irregular Choice shoes that Melissa simply could not live without, and once again it was back to the hotel to get changed and ready for lunch. I had bought a gorgeous coral pink skirt, a white cardigan with ¾ length sleeves and a pair of white shoes with flowers embroidered on them. I got dressed and looked in the mirror to be met by the reflection of my mother, circa 1960. Oh well, it had to happen one day.

Not exactly sure where the restaurant was, we decided to book a taxi to make sure we would not be late. And as usual in Dublin, the taxi driver was chatty and friendly. Like many Dubliners he has noticed the changes that have taken place I the city, and although grudgingly accepting that change is all part of life, he wasn't mad keen on the way in which the economy was going, the Celtic Tiger seemingly gone for a nap.

'There's one thing you'll never change about Dublin though,' I pointed out. 'The sense of humour, there's nowhere in the world with a sense of humour like Dublin.'

'That's true enough,' replied the driver. 'Shame we can't fucking sell it,' he added drolly, without looking back, and confirming my words with that one line.

The restaurant where we had agreed to meet was Dunne And Crescenzi on South Frederick Street, an aptly named place to meet the infamous Lee Dunne, and when the taxi pulled up outside, there he was, sitting waiting for us at a table outside the restaurant, his white hair glistening in the sunshine.

Although we had never met before in person, he knew who was heading towards him, and as we approached he got to his feet and smiled as he held out his arms in welcome to me. It was like being wrapped in the arms of an old friend, just as it should have been, and if I had any trepidation about meeting my mailing buddy, it was washed away with a kiss to the cheek and a hug that told me we shall always be friends. He then turned to Melissa and Jade, hugging them both in turn and a voice came from the other side of the street.

'Jesus! Lee Dunne, how do you do it?' A man asked in a loud voice. Lee laughed.

'I simply get up in the morning,' he replied; quick as a flash, in his easy, relaxed tone.

Inside the restaurant was like being transported to a little Italy where all the customers spoke with Irish accents. The staff were Italian, the food was wholly Italian, and every wall was lined from floor to ceiling with shelves that held a myriad of bottles of wine. The slogan for the restaurant could well have been 'You don't have to be good looking to work here, but it helps.'

Seated at a table just inside the door, Lee told us to choose whatever we wanted from the substantial menu. Of course Jade, on her eternal quest to discover the best lasagne in the world, chose lasagne. Melissa, ever eager in her quest to find the best salad in the world chose her meal from this part of the menu. I quite fancied

the ravioli, only ever having tried the tinned, Heinz variety up until then, but

unfortunately that was only on the evening menu. So, there I was, in one of the most

authentic Italian restaurants I had ever seen, ordering chicken and roast potatoes, in

keeping with the food philistine that I am. Lee had a salad and a bowl of minestrone

soup, and throughout the meal kept us entertained with anecdotes that enthralled. I

don't think I have ever known Jade to be so quiet as she soaked up every word that

Lee spoke that day, captivated by his stories.

We were not to be disappointed with our meeting with Lee Dunne. It was

no real surprise to find that over the past couple of years I had communicated with a

man who was exactly what I expected him to be. He is warm, intelligent, funny,

entertaining… and real, so very, very real.

Lee Dunne makes no excuses for his colourful past; his past is what made

him the man he is today. Yes he was a bit of a lad in years gone by, to say the least,

but without his past, Lee would not have developed the personality that now makes

him one of the finest people I have ever had the privilege to know.

All too soon two hours had gone by, we were eating desert and it was almost

time for us to go. I could quite happily have sat there another couple of hours until it

was teatime, and then a few more hours until it was time for an Italian breakfast, but

we had a concert to go to that night, and Lee had his writing and his beloved wife,

Maura, to get home to.

Outside the restaurant we said goodbye with hugs and kisses, and it was hard

to leave my pal. Lee is so much more to me than someone I write to; if I lived nearby

I know we would drop into one another's houses for coffee and that we would spend

time together as friends should. But there is a sea between us, so all we have is our letters. We parted, and my girls and I wiped tears from our eyes as we headed off back to the city.

At the bottom of Dame Street a woman played a harp, the haunting, beautiful music somehow blending with the roar of the passing traffic, and just across from her a man filled in the pavement with poetry written in coloured chalks, his way of making a living in a city where he could find no work. We crossed over Dame Street as the lights changed, and on into Westmorland Street.

There, next to a boarded up property, we came across Pat Ingoldsby selling his books of poetry. Pat was once involved with children's television in Ireland, but these days he is to be found selling his work to the passing public. The rat race is not for Pat; he is happy writing and selling his poetry, but most of all he is happy meeting the people who pass by. We stopped to talk and he asked us what we had been doing. It was nice to smile and tell him who we had just been to lunch with. We chatted for a while, and then we bought one of his books, which he gladly signed for me. I have read it from cover to cover, which is further than I ever got with the book of Byron poems I have upstairs, but then Byron is not quite so entertaining as Pat Ingoldsby.

We tried to have a nap that afternoon, in readiness for the concert that night, but it didn't happen for me. Since arriving in Dublin I had put my troubles as far to the back of my mind as I could, and all that was on my head that afternoon was going to my first concert in… so many years I hate to count.

The last person I saw in concert was Gene Pitney, back in 1980. And before that it was Gary Glitter. When I told this to my boss at work he grimaced at the mention of the glittery one's name.

'We didn't know what he was back then,' I pointed out to Harry.

'But didn't the costumes give you a clue?' Harry asked.

I remember the first time I ever saw Pink on TV. It's rare these days that an artist makes me sit up and listen, and there is so much wishy-washy crap in the charts that it all seems to blend into one commercialised track. So I had got to a stage when I used to record Top of the Pops, only listening to chosen tracks. Pink, Get the Party Started, was one such track. I played in through, rewound and played it again, rewound and played it again, then went online to find the album this song came from.

When the album arrived in the post I was not disappointed and Pink became one of those rare artists whose albums I bought one after the other. So going to see her live was so exciting that there was not a chance of my getting a nap that afternoon. If I thought of the upcoming treatment that had been filling my head for weeks, then it was only a fleeting thought that was cast out as I showered and got changed that evening.

It was a long walk to the O2, but the sun was shining, and we were in good company. We had been worried about not being able to find our way to the new arena, but it was easy, all we had to do was follow the crowds. People selling t-shirts, rabbit's ears that flashed (?), and all manner of Pink memorabilia (Mostly not official merchandise, but who cared?) lined the route and helped to build the air of anticipation along the way.

And then we were there, the huge building loomed above us and we joined the queue of excited concertgoers. I had been worried that I would be the oldest one there, but no, it appears that Pink appeals to all age groups, from little kiddies to grannies like me. We went inside and found our way to our seats easy enough. The O2 is huge, but it has been well laid out so that it is easy to find your way around. We were there early, and it would be a couple of hours yet before Pink would take to the stage. But that didn't matter. Jade was so excited I thought she was going to burst, and when the support act, Raygun, took to the stage she cheered and whooped like it was Pink herself.

By the time Pink was due on stage all the seats had been filled and the anticipation that buzzed around the arena was electrifying. Mysterious shapes behind the stage curtains added to the excitement. And suddenly there she was, being hoisted from a trapdoor in the stage, high into the air, as her music filled the arena.

The girl in front of Melissa leapt to her feet in excitement, almost as though her seat had been electrified. But this didn't deter Melissa from seeing the concert, and she simply took to her feet too, as did many people around us who were just way too excited to stay seated.

However, the woman who sat behind Melissa was not happy and declared in a loud voice that she had paid for her seat and couldn't see because Melissa was standing up. She sat there with a face like a slapped arse, moaning and whinging throughout the entire two-hour performance.

In spite of the fact that all around her people had got to their feet, this woman had paid for her seat and expected everyone around her to sit down. She was at a Pink concert, the atmosphere was electric, the excitement was rocket fuelled, but this woman expected everyone to stay seated as though they were at the Gaiety at a bloody pantomime.

She continued to whinge to such an extent that I thought Melissa was going to slap her at one stage. Melissa later told me that she had wanted to, but knowing that she would probably have been thrown out of the concert and possibly arrested made sure that she kept her hands to herself.

The woman left just before Pink came on stage to perform her spectacular encore; probably concerned that there could have been a confrontation if she had stayed to the end. And then the end came, and we joined the other concertgoers to make our way back up the quays towards the city, still feeling elated from the experience of seeing Pink live.

I would recommend to anyone facing radiotherapy and chemotherapy to try to get away somewhere for a few days before it starts. This trip to Dublin was, for me, a blessed relief from the worry and fretting over the upcoming treatment. It was only two and a half days, but it was two and a half days filled with things to take my mind off what I had to face when I got home.

The following morning Melissa knocked on my hotel room door to see if I was going down to breakfast. I had already been up several hours by the time she called for me and was showered and dressed, ready to make the most of the day we had left in Dublin. She couldn't speak because she had lost her voice after joining in so enthusiastically the night before, so she squeaked and pointed in the direction of the lift and I got what she meant.

After breakfast we went walking around Dublin for the last time for this visit. We went to Walton's music shop, a Mecca for Jade when she is in Dublin, then we walked back down O'Connell Street, around Trinity College, where Jade hopes to attend as a student one day, and off towards Grafton Street, heading for St Stephen's Green, an oasis in the middle of the city.

Half way up Grafton Street there was a statue that hadn't been there before. I noticed its tie blowing in the wind, a strange thing to have on any statue, and realised that this was a living sculpture. However, Melissa and Jade didn't notice and strolled towards it at a leisurely pace.

'Boo!' The living statue scared the living daylights out of them, and jump-started their hearts.

We found out way to St Stephen's Green and sat in the sunshine, watching the pigeons, wondering how so many of them had ended up with deformed feet, some with little more than stumps to hobble around on as they begged for scraps of food from anyone who sat on the benches where they lived.

Time was going too fast, and soon it was time to make our way back down to the hotel, where our suitcases were waiting to be taken to the airport, back to England, back to reality, back to the fear and dread that I had left behind for too short a period of time. But we had memories that would last forever, and although our trip to Dublin had been brief, I was so glad we had this time together. It was an expensive trip, but that didn't matter, what mattered was that I had a few days when my mind was not drowning in fear.

April 22nd 2009

Last night we landed at Manchester airport, I slept in my own bed for just one night and today I am going to Preston where the feeding tube is going to be fitted tomorrow.

If I am not totally honest in what I am writing here, then I will have failed not only myself but also any potential reader looking for the truth of his/her own situation. So, to be honest, today I am really scared. I woke up at 6 am, tried to get back off to sleep but it wasn't happening in spite of the fact that I feel so very tired. So I got up, emailed some friends, listened to Colm and Jim Jim on the radio, unpacked my case from the Dublin trip, packed a smaller case to take to Preston, and have spent the last three hours fighting a desperate urge to run away. Of course, I won't run away, but the urge is there nonetheless.

Fast-forward 3 days and the job is done.

I had to report to the oncology department before I presented myself to ward 3, where I would be staying while the PEG feeding tube was to be fitted. The reason for attending the oncology department was so that a senior nurse could explain the finer details of the chemotherapy that I would be having every Tuesday, just a small amount to back up the radiotherapy. Somehow I had managed to misinterpret what Dr Siva had said, I had thought that it was to be just one session of chemotherapy, but no, it was to be one session of chemotherapy every Tuesday for the six weeks of the treatment.

Sitting in the waiting room, waiting (appropriately) for the nurse, I felt like a fish out of water. I didn't fit in; for one thing I had the wrong colour hair. Everyone else in that room had grey hair of some variation; it was like a sea of dandelion clocks. There was a guy with long hair tied back in a pony tail, sporting gold earrings and wearing faded denims, but even he had hair that was streaked several shades of grey and silver. Nobody spoke, nobody made eye contact and nobody smiled. It was a horrible place to sit and wait.

Nurse Wurzell came out and introduced herself to me. No, I am not making that name up. She brought me into a little room where she told me what would happen every Tuesday. I shall turn up at 8.30 am and will be given an infusion of poison that will kill off any bad cells in my body. Unfortunately it will also kill off any good cells, but that's just tough. The treatment will take all day because they have to give me other drugs to make sure I don't vomit and they have to flush out my kidneys to make sure they don't suffer from the effects of the poison.

Nurse Wurzell is a caring professional; I could tell this even if she hadn't been wearing a nurse's uniform. Nurse Wurzell explains everything the patient needs to know with an expression of concern on her face that is bordering on comical. Her 'understanding' look is pained, and while I appreciate that she is simply trying to be sympathetic and empathetic, she really could smile a little more. I know that cancer is not a happy situation, but we were sitting in a room in a hospital, not an antechamber of a funeral director's.

Along with explaining what will happen when I show up for chemotherapy she also advised that I should use condoms as contraception throughout the treatment. Ha! Is she for real? I know I haven't read the book Crazy Sexy Cancer Tips, but if Nurse Wurzell thought I was likely to feel sexy over the coming weeks she was in dreamland.

No doubt over the coming weeks I am going to have a lot more dealings with Nurse Wurzell, and perhaps my initial opinion will alter somewhat as the weeks go on. I hope so, because at the moment I am a tad worried that I am going to find her overly sympathetic countenance bloody irritating. Wearing an expression that looks like she has taken on the weight of the world's problems is not one that I want to face every Tuesday morning; a smile would be so much better.

I left my interview with Nurse Wurzell with a whole heap of pamphlets that I have yet to read. She told me most of what was in them anyway; things like how I should avoid takeaways, an easy thing to do in the town I live in. Next stop, to report to ward 3.

There had been an emergency on ward 3 that afternoon. I don't know what the emergency was but it meant that the nurses were behind with their work, and as I was part of their work this meant that getting me admitted was subject to a delay of several hours; hours that I spent in the otherwise abandoned room that was laughingly called the TV room.

Ok, there was a TV in there, and it *was* switched on, but because the aerial didn't work it really should have been renamed 'the radio room' as all I could do was listen to the TV shows. Of the dozens of chairs in that room the only ones in use were the ones taken up by myself and Tom and by a couple of young Asian men, one of whom was also waiting for admission. Patients do not use this room at all generally, and why would they? It is a room with chairs in it, and because the television aerial doesn't work, the room is useless as anything other than a waiting room. Besides, most people chose to make use of the Patientline system next to their beds rather than watch TV in a room down the corridor.

Eventually I convinced Tom that he should go home. There was no point in both of us going mad while we tried to make out the fuzzy pictures that were supposed to accompany the soundtrack to an old episode of Frost, and besides, Molly was already going to be late getting her dinner and it wasn't fair that the dog should suffer the effects of ward 3's emergency.

After Tom left, one of the young men who were still waiting spoke to me.

'Are you being admitted?' He asked, in a local accent.

'Eventually,' I said; my patience was running out a little by this stage. 'Are you being admitted?' I asked him.

The young man explained that he wasn't being admitted but his cousin was. He went on to explain that his cousin was having an operation to remove glands from his neck, that his cousin didn't speak any English, and that he had come over from Pakistan from the operation.

Was he being treated as a private patient? Does our NHS system now cover people in Pakistan? These are questions I could not bring myself to ask, but you have to wonder.

Eventually I was signed in and allocated a bed in a bay that contained 3 other patients. Next to my bed was a woman who had been through a boob job; I don't know if this was cosmetic or for medical reasons; well, it's not polite to ask. Across from her was a teenager who I presumed was in to have her mobile phone surgically removed from her hand. Even when she was eating and drinking the phone was never put down. Opposite me was an old lady I will call Mavis, not her real name.

If Mavis is anything to go by, The Who got it right when they said 'Hope I die before I get old' in their song 'My Generation'. I know there are many old people out there who are in fine fettle in their 80s and beyond, but not so in the case of Mavis. She sat up in bed, but only because many pillows propped her up, otherwise she wouldn't have had the mental ability to think about getting into a sitting position. She couldn't walk, not even with the help of a walking frame, she couldn't feed herself, and while she was capable of speech she was incapable of conversation because her mind simply could not cope with the complexities of social dialogue exchange. She had to wear a 'pad', which was really a large nappy, because she was doubly incontinent. If Mavis had been a dog she would have been put to sleep a long time ago, because it would be considered cruel to keep a dog alive with such lack of dignity and with no quality of life whatsoever. But human beings do not have this choice. Human beings are not allowed the dignity of humanity. Mavis didn't know her family, Mavis didn't know where she was nor why she was there, and neither do I.

Yet the nurses at Preston treated Mavis with the respect and dignity any human being deserves. They didn't get annoyed when she snapped at them, they didn't lose patience when she refused to eat or drink, and even when her nappy smelled like the sewers of London they put on a brave face, took a deep breath, and cleaned her up to make her comfortable again. Comfort is all Mavis has now, and those young girls were happy to see that she had it in abundance.

This care was something I witnessed and experienced several times at Preston hospital. Having attended many hospitals in my lifetime, it's only fair to point out here that the medical staff at Preston hospital are the kindest, most caring, understanding medical staff I have ever met.

Mavis's granddaughter came to visit that afternoon.

'Who are you?' Mavis demanded of her in an angry tone. 'I don't know who you are.' She snapped, and eventually the granddaughter left, wiping away her tears as she headed off down the corridor. Mavis didn't notice she had left, and probably didn't remember her ever being there.

There's not much point in trying to get an early night in hospital. It's not really possible to get to sleep until the nurses have finished their final rounds of taking blood pressure, checking temperatures and handing out drugs. So instead I watched TV, caught the latest episode of Desperate Housewives and then settled down to a peaceful night's sleep, thanks to the earplugs that I always have the good sense to bring into hospital with me. I woke the next morning with some trepidation about the procedure that was going to take place that day, but what bothered me more than the anticipation of the small operation was the fasting. In spite of my apprehension, I woke up hungry.

As I said earlier, breakfast at Preston hospital is particularly good, and they serve up the creamiest porridge I have ever tasted. No hotel has ever dished up such smooth oatmeal as the kitchens at Preston manage to present. I was hungry, and thirsty, but I would not be allowed to break my fast until four hours after the procedure had taken place. Once four hours had passed I would be allowed some water, and if I managed to keep that down they would let me have something to eat. So, when I was still waiting to go down for the procedure at lunch time I got the dinner lady to put an egg mayonnaise sandwich on brown bread into the ward fridge for me, with my name on it. It was something to look forward to later.

A porter turned up late in the morning, complete with a wheelchair that held my bulging records folder. This was it; I was off to have a feeding tube fitted to my tummy, and my tummy wasn't at all happy going by the way it recoiled in horror at the prospect. But like so much I have had to face lately, it was a case of getting on with it. I did feel particularly ridiculous at having to be wheeled there when I had two perfectly good legs to walk on.

I say 'perfectly good legs' but I have to confess to some cellulite in that area. However, they do the job they are intended for; the hold me up and propel me in whichever direction I need to go. But the porter explained that it is 'hospital policy' for patients to be transported from one department to another in this way, something to do with being sued if I had an accident while walking.

I thought back to when I had my two operations, and how each time I had walked alongside a nurse to the operating rooms, never once having fallen over something, and even if I had, would I have considered suing the NHS for not transporting me in a wheelchair? Of course I wouldn't. The NHS may have its failings here and there but, compared to many countries of the world, the system of medical care in the UK is, in my humble opinion, something to be cherished, not vilified.

The wheelchair trundled along corridors, into the lift, up or down... not sure which (but does it matter) and along more corridors until we reached a department that I recognised. Unless they were going to carry out the procedure in radiotherapy… I realised that I was here to have my mask verified, and that the fitting of the feeding tube would happen later in the day.

The porter parked the wheelchair in the same area that I had waited in when I had come to have my mask fitted. Around me, other patients waited, and suddenly I didn't feel quite so bad about my own cancer as I noticed a young man who had his nose removed. He waited with his wife and little girl, seemingly happy in spite of his nose being replaced by bandages and plasters. Again I wondered; if there were a God, why would He be so cruel to this young family? Why would He not intervene to make this man whole again?

The waiting area was full of people, some wearing bad wigs, some with hair that made me wonder. Mostly the people who waited were elderly, and while I am in my fifties, I felt young amongst them.

I didn't have long to wait before my name was called, and much to the surprise of those seated around me I stood up out of the wheelchair as though a miracle had just taken place. I was shown into the radiotherapy room where the mould for the mask had been made, and the mask, now hardened, was placed on my face to make sure it fitted snugly, as it is designed to hold my head still while I am blasted with radiation. My eyes closed automatically as it came over my face, and once closed and the mask is clipped in place it is not possible to open them again. I don't like not being able to see what is happening, not that it really matters, as I can't make a difference to the processes by *seeing* what is going on. The radiologists seemed to be putting stickers here and there on the mask, and it didn't take long for them to be happy with whatever it was they were doing and I was freed from the restraints of the mask.

Another feeling I don't like is the mask being clipped into place and held fast. Even if I wanted to, even if I *had* to, I would not be able to move once I am fixed to the table by the mask that covers my face.

After the verification of the mask I was asked to wait at the seating area again as a nurse needed to have a word with me about the impending treatment. There were only two men sitting there now, talking animatedly about rugby, and while I would have loved to have had a conversation with someone, anyone, about anything that wasn't radiotherapy, my knowledge of rugby is limited to the names of a few international players, Irish ones at that; would they have been impressed that I knew who Ronan O'Gara is?

Dr Siva went past, and stopped to say hello. He's a likeable man with great teeth. I don't mean great as in big, I mean great as in beautifully white, the kind of teeth that can light up a face when it smiles. And as I said earlier, Dr Siva has a nice smile.

'Hi... how was Dublin?' He asked me, and I told him it had been wonderful. It was nice to have him stop and speak to me like that; it made me feel less of a number and more of a person that he remembered me. Remembering me transcribed into caring about me.

I can't remember the name of the nurse who took me off into a small room to give me a sheet of paper containing revised dates and times that I was to have my treatments. And even though it was only a couple of days ago, I can recall little of the conversation I had with her. Other than her advice on makeup:

She told me that if I wanted to wear foundation I should not do so any further down my face than just below my cheekbones. Now how weird would that look? It's bad enough when women take their foundation to the chin and forget they have a neck, but to take it to half way down the face and leave the bottom half… well, that's just downright silly. No, I'm not going to bother with foundation at all. I'll put my eyes on, but the uneven skin tone on the face is just going to have to remain unrectified during the process of the treatment.

I was taken back out to reception, where I was left sitting in my wheelchair and told to wait for the porter to take me back to the ward, where the anticipation of the fitting of the feeding tube began to turn into a panic inside my head that would not allow me to concentrate on anything. I know I watched the Jeremy Kyle show on TV that afternoon, but I haven't got a clue what it was about; although I assume it was all to do with DNA tests to find out of Daz was the father of Jazz's baby, and/or lie detector results.

'Lynn Connolly?' Another porter arrived on the ward at about 4.00 pm. By which time I was seriously hungry and thirsty, and my anxiety levels were going through the roof.

'Never heard of her,' I quipped. Why do I always do that? When other people are scared and anxious they behave like scared, anxious people, whereas I have to crack jokes as though I am there to audition for Live at the Apollo.

'I can tell it's you, the fear on your face is a dead giveaway,' the porter replied and I gave in and allowed my bed to be wheeled through the corridors and down in the lift to the endoscope department. Being taken to the department in my bed seemed to make the whole event more serious than it would if I were taken there in a wheelchair. Even when I went for operations I walked to the operating theatres under my own steam, so it worried me that I was being taken to have the feeding tube fitted on my bed.

I was seriously scared, even though I had been assured that the sedation would make sure I knew nothing about the procedure afterwards, I had been told that just for a split second I would feel a choking sensation as the endoscope passed down my throat, and this is what was making me very nervous indeed. I had been told that I wouldn't feel the hole being made in my tummy for the tube to pass through, so this wasn't my main concern, no, it was the choking thing I didn't like the idea of.

Inside the department several nurses gave me more assurances that I would be fine, it would be over before I knew it and I wouldn't remember a thing. And little by little I began to feel a tiny bit better about what I was about to go through.

A man in the bed opposite mine was recovering from his procedure before he was to be allowed home, and he assured me that it was easy, that he had had a camera put down and he had hardly felt a thing, he said that the procedure had been uncomfortable, but not painful. It was much later that I realised this man had a camera put up his nostril; the same procedure that I had done every month since my last operation. But at the time his words were something of a comfort to me, and I tried very hard not to panic.

There was a bout a twenty-minute wait before my bed was wheeled into a room that resembled the ones where general anaesthesia is administered prior to an operation. John Pendlebury introduced himself, and while he didn't introduce himself as 'Dr' I assume this to be his title as he was about to administer the sedation and carry out the procedure. He told me again that I would be heavily sedated throughout the procedure. He injected liquid antibiotic into the cannula that had been fitted to the back of my hand a few hours earlier, and then administered the sedation. But if I had expected to find myself drifting off to sleep I was in for a shock.

A black plastic tube, resembling a vacuum cleaner attachment, was placed in my mouth and the endoscope was pushed through this and down my throat. Yes I felt like I was choking, I felt like I was having a golf club shoved down my throat (not that I have ever had a golf club shoved down my throat by way of comparison) as the endoscope guided the feeding tube towards my stomach in a way that I can only describe as vicious and brutal.

Now I found out why there were so many nurses in the room, they were there to hold me down as I fought like a wild cat trapped in a net against the onslaught of the feeding tube and the endoscope. Had the nurses not been there I have no doubt that I would have tried to pull the scope back out and I would most certainly have punched the doctor, probably would have knocked him out.

I felt the slit being made in my stomach, I felt the tube being pulled through it and I felt the tube being clipped into place. In short, I felt it all! I have been through some painful experiences in my life, but never have I gone through anything so truly horrific as having the PEG fitted that day.

When it was over the Dr calmly wheeled his chair over into the corner and had his back to me as they wheeled my bed back out of the room as he completed his paperwork. I'd love to see what he wrote there. He never even bothered his arse to say 'sorry' as I was wheeled out. I so hope that was the last time I ever see that man, or I could end up having a few words to say to him that he might not want to hear.

I am sure I did not receive enough sedation that day, and I don't feel as though the time and care was taken to make sure of this. I could be wrong, I'm no doctor, but it seems that my experience of having the feeding tube fitted is quite unique.

Since then I have researched the subject on the Internet and I cannot find one person who had the same experience that I suffered that day. I seem to be the only one who felt, and remembers, every moment of the dreadful incident that I still fail to see as anything other than the trauma it was.

I hold John Pendlebury wholly responsible for this. As a doctor it was up to him to ensure that the correct level of sedation was administered. In all the time I spent at Preston hospital, this was the only individual I met who, frankly, didn't give a fuck what pain he caused.

And afterwards, well, I had been told that the tube would feel 'a little uncomfortable'. Sorry, a little uncomfortable is needing a cushion at your back while sitting on the sofa watching TV. What I went through after having the tube fitted was agonising pain. OK, this was probably due to the fact that I had fought so fiercely during the procedure; no doubt there had been more muscle damage than there would normally be because of this. But I wouldn't have fought so hard if I had been sedated like I had been assured I would be; like everyone else says they were.

I was in pain when I got back to the ward, but I was still hungry, yet I had four hours to wait before I could even be given a small amount of water to drink. I was thirsty, but all I was allowed was a stick with a bit of moist cotton wool on the end, and this did little to relieve the thirst that made me feel as though I were in the middle of a desert, far away from the nearest oasis. But eventually the four hours was up, I was allowed water to drink, and as soon as the nurses were happy I had kept this down one of them went to get me my sandwich… only to find that it was gone!

What kind of miserable bastard takes a sandwich from a fridge that a fasting patient has put away? My name was on it for God's sake! All I can say is that I hope the thieving git who stole my sandwich that day is hungry themselves one day.

A nurse kindly made me some toast, but as ever in hospitals, there was not enough butter on it. Still, I was grateful for even this small offering, as I had gone over twenty-four hours with nothing to eat.

I was given painkillers to help me through the night, and although my stomach was still feeling the effects of the invasion I managed to get off to sleep with the help of liquid dihydrocodeine and Paracetamol.

I woke up in the middle of the night, needing to cough but in too much pain to do so, much like I had been when I had my hysterectomy. I reached out for my cup of water, desperate for it to stem the tickle in my throat, but I missed it and knocked it onto the floor. I couldn't hold the cough in, but when it came it also brought with it a sharp pain in my stomach where the tube had been inserted.

I pressed the emergency button for help, expecting a nurse to respond quickly, but nobody came and I coughed again, bringing another wave of pain to my stomach. So I pressed the button again, and again. But nobody came. Perhaps they were busy with an emergency, I don't know. All I know is that eventually I was verbally pleading for help and that it was the elderly lady in the bed next to mine (the boob job lady having gone home earlier) who responded to my plea and she retrieved my cup and helped me into a sitting position to drink from it.

Eventually a nurse appeared, and she got me some more pain relief so that I could sleep the rest of the night in relative comfort.

I wonder, is this a difference between private and NHS care? Do private patients get priority treatment when emergency buttons are pressed?

I hadn't looked at the tube. I didn't want to see it yet. But the following day I suddenly felt very wet around my right side and went into a bit of a panic. There were nurses on the ward already, and when I told them I was all wet for no apparent reason they sprang into action.

The tube that comes out of the tummy has a clip half way down, and at the end of it there is a cannula type fixture. In this case the clip was open, the cannula had come open too, and the wetness I was feeling was the contents of my stomach being drained away. Oh Yuck!

The nurses quickly put the plug back into place on the cannula and helped me to get changed into clean clothes. It was an unpleasant experience, but at least it made me look at the tube and become familiar with the way it worked.

I was allowed home on the Friday, only because I managed to do an Oscar winning performance on the pain front. I was still in more pain than I should have been, but because I managed to convince the medical staff otherwise I was allowed home. I needed to spend the weekend in my own home before the treatment started.

But if I were expecting the pain from the tube insertion to die down over the next couple of days, I was to be disappointed as the pain and discomfort continued as my treatment began.

27th April 2009

Today was my first day of radiotherapy and I can't say I felt particularly scared about the event. Yes it was a little daunting, going there alone, travelling a 140 mile round trip and going through the treatment itself, although I had been assured that the treatment itself is totally painless, it is the effects of the treatment that cause problems.

My driver for the day was Tony, a lovely man from Blackburn (he hadn't travelled up from Blackburn specially, he had moved here some years ago) and I had to sit in the back of the car because the front seat was taken up by a lady who needed some room for her prosthetic leg. She told me how it had been rubbing, and had become very sore, and so she was going to see a specialist to try to resolve the problem. But she didn't tell me how she had ended up with a prosthetic leg, and I didn't ask, and I still want to know!

Arriving at Preston, I presented myself at the reception desk, minus my list of treatment dates because nobody had told me that I needed to bring this with me. No matter, the receptionist wrote my name on a piece of paper, handed it back to me and said:

'LA5.'

Which was completely meaningless to me, other than it could have been half of a Lancaster postcode.

'LA5?' I repeated in question.

'Machine number 5,' the receptionist said, as though this would make it all perfectly clear. It didn't. I shook my head to indicate that I didn't have the vaguest idea what she was talking about, and she explained that the machines were numbered, and that the machine I would be treated on was to be number 5; LA5 standing for Linear Amplifier number 5. The only time I had heard the words 'linear amplifier' before was in relation to a device that made a CB radio work better as it boosted the signal. She pointed me in the right direction, and off I went, still feeling that I shouldn't really be there. I wonder if this is a feeling that is going to perpetuate until the very end of the treatment.

I was entitled to a free hot drink; tea, coffee or hot chocolate (with marshmallows if so required), but I wasn't sure how long the wait would be to be called in for treatment, so I decided to get a bottle of water instead. I took a seat at the café style waiting area, but decided to forego on the Caravan Club magazines that seemed to be on every table. I wasn't the only one alone; some were alone, some were with partners, some were with carers, but I felt like the only one who had nobody to talk to, even though that was obviously not the case as there were quite a few solitary people there that morning.

Oh dear, that sounds so sad, but that's how I felt, alone, lonely, and yes, a little sad. The woman I had shared the car with on my visit to have the mask made had told me that she had met some lovely people at the department, and that I would find that there was always someone to talk to. So maybe it is just me, and perhaps I am in some way anti-social, but I didn't find anyone there to strike up a conversation with.

Some women wore wigs to cover up their baldness, and some of these wigs should have been discarded to a bin a long time previous. I'm not going to single out individual cases where the wigs were obvious, but I find it hard to believe that anyone could look in the mirror and think 'Nobody will know.' when the wigs in question were... well, very *much* in question.

There is a particular style of free NHS wig that seems very popular, a blonde bob with a fringe (bangs) that has been nicely coloured and shaped. However, as this style of wig is the most popular, the resulting parade of 'Doris Day through the ages' is more than a little amusing.

There are two notice boards in the waiting area of LA5, and both are completely covered by Thank You cards that have been sent in by grateful patients. I wonder if I will do the same at the end of my treatment, after all it seems a nice thing to do. At the centre of one of these boards there is a card that has been made especially for the occasion of someone surviving radiotherapy; and whoever made it really could have tried to make it a bit more cheerful. The card is four times the size of a normal sized greetings card, and is made from dark brown card that has been decorated with gold lettering. Somebody has gone to an awful lot of trouble to make sure their card stands out, but it does so for all the wrong reasons. It is dark and gloomy, it takes up far too much of the notice board and it looks as though it has been made by a 5 year old. Oh dear, now I have probably upset someone.

Anushka, a girl I took to straight away, came out and called my name. Sometimes we have to take a while to decide whether or not we like someone; but not so in the case of Anushka, who introduced herself and informed me that although her name is Russian, she isn't. She also has a rather exotic surname, and I must make a point of finding out why she is so called. Anushka is one of the girls who work on LA5, and although I have been introduced to some of the others it is only she whose name I have remembered and put to a face.

'Can I just check your date of birth and your address please Lynn?' Anushka asked. 'We need to be sure we have the right person,' she explained.

'Why; just in case some crazy person has wandered in off the street and decided to take this treatment for me?' I smiled at her as the nervous quip fell out of my mouth, in the way that they do when I am nervous or under pressure.

The treatment on day one followed the pattern that is going to be set for every weekday for the next 6 weeks. I lay on the cold, metal table, the mask was placed on my face and clipped into place, and then the girls set about saying numbers. I gather this is to measure exactly where the rays will be directed. I didn't ask because it's rather irrelevant. Then the girls leave the room, the machine starts whirring and buzzing, and a couple of CD tracks later they are back and unclipping the mask to set me free.

However, this first day was the only day I listened to Andy Williams; the following day I made sure I had some CDs of my own to choose from.

The treatment itself is not remotely painful and is over fairly quickly, but for anyone who suffers from claustrophobia it must be a rather traumatic experience when the mask is clipped into place. The mask is hard, it follows the contours of the head and neck and when it is clipped into place movement is not possible.

I must stress that this in only for cancers of the head and neck. Anyone with cancer in a different part of the body will not have this facemask made. I haven't asked, but I'm sure that when treating cancers such as prostate cancer there is no mould made of that part of the body.

The trick is to relax, and anyone who thinks they may suffer from the effects of claustrophobia really needs to discuss this with their consultant before treatment starts, so that some plan can be made in order to help the patient relax. If this is a need for tranquilliser of some sort then so be it, whatever gets you through it. The treatment is so much more important than getting over a panic attack. I am in no way belittling panic attacks here because I once suffered from them myself and I know how awful they can be. My first one was a heart attack, or so I thought at the time, and my second happened in the middle of Debenhams and I couldn't find my way out of the store. So if you do feel that you would suffer from being held tightly in place while the treatment is being carried out then I suggest you get this sorted out before treatment begins. Yes the radiologists can get you out of there in a matter of seconds, all you have to do is raise your hand and they are right by your side, but then the treatment has to start all over again, so it really is best to get it over with without going into a panic.

Tuesday 28th April

First day of chemotherapy, and like with everything I have gone through with this illness I had no notion of what I was going to face. I had to be up at 5.00 am because my driver was coming for me at 5.50. There were other people to pick up along the way, firstly a man from Barrow, who sat in the front seat while his leg and arm went into the boot. No he was not particularly tall; he was just one of many people I was to meet over the coming weeks who have had limbs severed for one reason or another. Next we had to pick up another man from Ulverston who turned out to be a head and neck surgeon himself, suffering from a rare blood disorder that meant he could no longer work unless the treatment he is receiving works for him. We forget that doctors get sick too.

We arrived outside the Oncology department just after 8.00 am, early for my 8.30 appointment, but there was already someone working behind the desk and Barry, the porter I was later to find out works tirelessly in the department, was already setting up the tea bar for patients and putting out the daily newspapers in the waiting room; it's been ages since I read a daily paper so I scanned through the Sun while I was waiting, either for someone else to arrive or to be called into the treatment room. I was the only one there for some time, and once again my fight or flight instinct was kicking in, telling me (insanely) that I had a credit card in my bag, I could go to Manchester airport, get on a plane and go wherever I wanted to get away from this. But of course I couldn't get away from this; 'this' was inside me, 'this' was not going to go away just because I was in a different country. Besides, my passport was in drawer of the dresser in my dining room.

A couple came in, I gathered they were father and daughter and I thought it wonderful that she was being so supportive to her dad. From the outset Val was attentive to Eddie, offering to get him a drink, popping out to the shops to get him papers or whatever else he needed. They were both well dressed, but in a casual way, and I really should have copped on to the matching Lacoste trainers and the way they looked at one another. I was to find out a little later that Val and Eddie were not father and daughter but devoted husband and wife, so much so that it warms my heart just to think of them together even now. Yes there was an age gap, of some 20 years, but it didn't matter, I have rarely come across a couple so united in everything they do as this pair, and as time went on it was to become a privilege to know them both.

Eddie started his treatment on the same day as me, we are both having aggressive radiotherapy to both sides of the neck and chemotherapy every Tuesday, so Eddie and Val are going to be part of my life for some weeks to come; which is cool, I like them both. I love the way Eddie tells rude jokes in a voice that is a little too loud and Val looks at him in horror and tells him to shush as he chuckles. I love the way Val loves the colour pink and loves to draw pretty things to pass the time. They are such real people.

Nurse Alison called me in to the treatment room. I really must find out what her second name is, after all it's on her nametag. Alison is really nice, she has a smiling face, twinkling eyes, and a distinct sense of mischief that tells me she would probably be rather good fun on a night out. I couldn't see any sign of Nurse Wurzell, and the thought crossed my mind that she may be wearing a spare head.

I didn't expect the room to be as big as it is. It's about the size of a small school hall. The walls of one side of the room are lined with comfortable, recliner chairs where the patients sit while the chemotherapy drugs (or poisons) are slowly dripped into the veins with the help of blue machines that are attached to drip stands. Once attached to this machine and stand it is with you throughout the day.

Alison... I asked her if her name was spelt with an I or a Y. It would have been quite uncanny if it had been a Y, and yet I still felt a connection to my friend Alyson... almost as though she were there with me, holding the hand that Alison was not putting a needle into, and telling me I will be fine. (My friend Alyson died almost a year ago, cancer that had not been detected in her native South Africa was found to be right through her body when she moved to Russia, ironically to start a new life with her husband. It was too late for Alyson to be given chemotherapy, or radiotherapy.)

While Alison was putting the cannula into the back of my left hand, another lady was having the same thing done to her in the chair beside me. I couldn't help noticing that her name was Ann Smith, the same name as my sister-in-law. And once again I was reminded of someone who would happily have been there holding my hand if she could. But Ann lives in Cavan, and while I know she would be happy to be there for me, commuting from Cavan once a week would be rather impractical. But it was nice to be reminded of her just the same.

'This is the anti-sickness drug that I'm giving you first,' Alison explained as she attached a large syringe to the back of my hand. 'This makes sure that the treatment doesn't make you feel sick,' she added. 'But it does make you feel a bit funny as it goes in.'

'Funny; funny in what way?' I asked, feeling quite alarmed as all kinds of scenarios of 'feeling funny' ran through my head; sick, dizzy, nauseous... what?

'Like sitting on nettles,' she said, and I became even more alarmed as I couldn't see any dock leaves anywhere around. 'And the feeling might go up into your other bits too,' Alison added, and my feelings of alarm turned into almost panic.

Then the feeling hit, and I wanted to jump up out of the chair, but I knew there was no point to doing so as the feeling didn't come from the chair, it was deep inside me, and I know my eyes popped when Alison smiled and said 'It hit then?' amused, but not taking perverse pleasure from my discomfort. But then it started to go away as quickly as it had come, and on a scale of one to ten, I would count it as a four in the realms of surprises.

Then Alison attached up a large bag of saline to the drip stand, she set the pump working and I was guided over to one of the comfortable chairs where I would spend the next 5 hours. First the saline drip would flush through my system, then the chemotherapy (in my case, cisplatin) would be put into my drip, and then the saline drip would be repeated to flush through my kidneys again to make sure that the chemo didn't do any damage to them.

Ann and I were seated side by side and the day was to prove to be not nearly as bad as I thought it would be, mainly due to her company and the company of Val and Eddie. We talked for the next five hours, never seeming to run out of subject matter, although most of it seemed to centre around our treatments, how well we hoped to recover and what we intended to do afterwards. Ann is heading off on a mini-cruise to Ireland at the end of May, calling at Dublin first, so when she asked me for a list of my favourite restaurants in Dublin, and my favourite places to go while I'm there, I happily provided her with the names of several eateries, including Flanagan's in O'Connell Street, and Gallagher's Boxty House in Temple Bar, and told her not to miss out on the Kilmainham Jail tour. (Sitting here writing this now, the anticipation of going to Dublin again next year, of sampling my favourite restaurants... no, even that won't get the saliva flowing properly, so great is my anxiety.)

An Asian couple came into the room and the wife took her place to have her drugs attached to her cannula; her cannula was of the type that is permanently fitted for the duration of the treatment and her familiarity with the process was telling that she was already well into her treatment and knew exactly what to expect when she came into the room. Although the treatment takes around 5 hours, her husband sat with her throughout the whole time, not talking, just being there, and somehow it didn't seem to matter that they were not chatting, not even to one another, he was there, and it was obvious that he was there because he wanted to be, not because he had to be, and once again my heart was warmed by strangers.

Sonia... ah, what can I say about Sonia? She is a volunteer in the department, an unpaid assistant who is there every day to fetch and carry for the people who are undergoing treatment. Sonia gets drinks and snacks for people, dishes out lunch when the trolley comes around and talks to those who are there on their own so that they are not lonely. Sonia generally makes herself so useful that I can imagine the nurses would really miss her if she were not there. Sonia is not the fittest of people, having had major surgery herself in the past she rather struggles to get around, but that doesn't stop her from making sure that all of the patients have everything they need while she is there. Again... heart-warming.

At one point of the day Ann, Sonia and myself had a rather irreverent conversation about funerals, we all decided that the cost of these affairs are overpriced, and we laughed heartily at the shock on Sonia's face when I informed her that you can hire coffins these days. OK, maybe you had to be there, but it really was funny at the time, especially considering where we were having this conversation.

One thing that surprised me in the chemo department was how healthy most people looked. I had been dreading having to sit there for all that time surrounded by emaciated people with no hair. But that simply was not the case, and with most people in that room nobody would have guessed for a moment that they were ill at all.

On a shelf there were several brightly coloured helmets, and I later found out that these were used to attempt to prevent hair loss in patients receiving particular kinds of chemo, mainly the ones used in the treatment of breast cancer, by cooling the head before, during and after treatment. A young woman came into the treatment room later in the day; her hair was wispy and bald in patches, and to see her have one of the helmets fitted to her head as she sat down was a pitiful sight. I don't know how effective these helmets are, but on that young woman... what can I say, it just wasn't working and came across as clutching at straws.

To see young people being given chemotherapy was the hardest of all for me. It didn't seem fair that they had to go through this treatment when they should be off doing what other young people were. They should be working, socialising, shopping, having fun in general, not sitting in a hospital while poison was being pumped through their veins to kill of the invading cancers that they suffered from.

Ann's wig was great, a short blonde one with gold and red highlights, and unlike the Doris Day variety, I never would have known it was a wig if she hadn't told me. Of course, as soon as someone tells you they are wearing a wig you try to imagine what they would look like if they were not wearing it... generally unsuccessfully.

My treatment finished before the others that day, and saying goodbye to everyone before I left to go to the radiotherapy department was something of a wrench that I hadn't expected. I didn't know whether to lean down and hug my companions, or just to say cheerio. There was something a bit too final about the hug thing; after all, none of us were planning on dying any day soon, so I just left with a 'See you again.' As I was pretty sure I would.

Passing by the Asian couple, the wife looked at me and said 'bye'. And there was I thinking that she hadn't even noticed my existence. She even managed a little smile. I was reminded of the scene from One Flew over a Cuckoo's nest when the native American guy says 'thanks' to Jack Nicholson when he hands him a piece of gum; the only word the character speaks up until that point.

Before I left I was given tablets to give me an appetite (steroids), and tablets to ward of sickness, and then I was off to find my way through the maze of corridors through the hospital to the radiotherapy department for my second bout of treatment. I got there for about 3.00 pm, and as I sat waiting for my name to be called I experienced the most dreadful loneliness I have ever known in my life. All around me people sat waiting, either for their own treatment or for their loved ones to complete theirs. I was surrounded by people, and yet I was alone, horribly alone in a way I have never known before. I don't normally have a problem with my own company; loneliness is not something I normally suffer from, as I can usually simply get lost in my own thoughts if I have nothing more to do. But there in that waiting room I was engulfed with sadness; and a sense of solitude that I had never known before.

Bringing in my own CDs to be played during the treatment was a great idea, and when my name was finally called I decided there was only one man who could soothe my senses while I lay on that cold table with machines buzzing around me, and that man had to be Eminem, much to the surprise of the radiotherapist who took the CD from me with a raised eyebrow. 'Loose Yourself' is a song that can always raise me up out of dark moments. I'm not saying it would work for everyone but when

Eminem says 'Lose yourself in the music, the moment, you own it, you better never let it go; You only get one shot, do not miss this chance to blow, 'cos opportunity comes once in a lifetime…' And at the end of the track when he says 'You can do anything you set your mind to man.' Well for me his words are uplifting, and offer the listener belief in the self. I wouldn't expect it to effect everyone in the same way, but most people have a song like Lose Yourself, a song that will bring them out of the doldrums in most situations. So take your own music into treatment, be it The Sound of Music or Eminem… it doesn't matter what it takes to get you through. I intend to slowly go through my CD collection, and each day I'm planning to discover artists I have not listened to in ages, and the radiotherapists, probably, have not heard of at all, until now. People like Millie Jackson, Aslan, Grace Jones… they are all going to help me to come through this thing, even if they don't know it.

I wonder what a group consisting of Millie Jackson, Aslan, Grace Jones and Eminem would sound like.

The rest of the week went by without any hitches. On a couple of days we had to pick up a gentleman who lives in a gorgeous little cottage near Grange, which added considerable time onto the journey, but not in a bad way, the country roads are pretty, Grange is a lovely village, and there's not much point in getting stressed out about minor delays. After all, the gentleman in question actually lives closer to the hospital than I do, and nobody complains about me getting picked up first.

My first weekend off treatment was spent in catching up on correspondence. I had intended to do a lot of copy/paste work on the emails to my friends to let them know how I was getting on, but when it came to writing the letters I found I couldn't do it that way because it would have been like cheating. Each one of my friends care about me, and it's the least I can do to give them individual time at the weekend.

I am so grateful for the care and love I am surrounded by, and cannot imagine how hard all of this would be for someone who is alone with the process. My family and friends exude love without having to say so, and I feel very privileged to be cocooned in this way. I know there is not one of my family or friends who would not drop everything to be by my side if that was my wish, and if I can't spend a bit of time writing to them as individuals, well, what a sad friend I would be. Hence, keeping in touch, and letting everyone know how I was getting on took up most of that first Saturday off. Later a trip to the supermarket, where I chose some foodstuff that I knew I was going to enjoy that weekend, even if food wouldn't taste quite so good in the future. This was a time to spoil myself, and so I chose my favourite foods to eat that weekend. Had I been able to see into the future, I would probably have spent every waking moment eating.

4th May 2009

Today is a Bank holiday, for anyone who is working or in school. But for me it is business as usual and I have to go to Preston for another dose of radiotherapy. It's only been a week, and although up until now I couldn't have said I felt any effects from the treatment, today I am definitely feeling something is going on, something not quite right, or something right if you take into account that certain things are *supposed* to happen, like a dry mouth, which I am suffering from at night time only at the moment, but I know that will extend as time goes on, and I have to say I am not exactly looking forward to it.

I woke up this morning with a mouth like a camel's armpit. I'm not sure if that statement is technically correct, for all I know a camel's armpit may be rather moist, but my throat was totally dry, my tongue had a strange white coating all over it and my throat is a tad sore. When I say a tad sore, I mean it hurts a little, nothing to whinge about.

I also have diarrhoea (spelt right first time), and I'm not sure that is normal. When I gave in and started using the painkillers I knew I also had to take something for the constipation that would occur as a result of taking dihydrocodeine, so I started taking Movicol, which is apparently a lot gentler than senna. Whether or not I have taken too much Movical (which I stopped taking 2 days ago) or whether the diarrhoea is as a result of something else… who knows? I will tell them about it at Preston when I get there today. I think it might be an idea to take a change of clothing just to be on the safe side. Diarrhoea waits for no man… or woman. And as my stomach is currently making noises more usually associated with Darth Vader's light sabre, I don't think it's quite settled down as yet.

I had thought (see what thought did) that Bank Holiday Monday would mean that the motorway would be relatively calm. Wrong! Not only was the road nose to tail with vehicles, every second vehicle had a caravan or a trailer tent attached to the back of it. It was pouring with rain, which is probably why the majority of campers/caravaners decided to go home early, and as most of them were heading south, the motorway we had to travel on was particularly busy. The journey to Preston normally takes about an hour and a half, but today it took nearer to two hours because of the people who believe that it's fun to tow a tin box on wheels half way around the country rather than pay a hotel bill, or even a B&B.

Of course, the roads were even more congested by the people who take their children out for the day to drive up and down the motorway, the highlight of their day being a stop off at Burger King. When our kids were little we used to take them to the beach, the zoo, out to the country… never once do I recall heading for a motorway service station in promise of a great day out.

Once there, many of these unimaginative parents seem to forget that they brought the children there I the first place, going by the way the kids run around yelling and screaming while their parents tuck into their Whoppas, oblivious to the fact that their offspring are annoying other grown ups. I can't begin to imagine how many children's meals are sold at Burger King service station outlets on Bank holidays. Apart from the poor kid whose parents cared so much for his nutritional input that they had kindly bought him a cold pasta salad from M&S. Boy was he disappointed by his day trip to the motorway.

I was half way through my double bacon cheeseburger when I suddenly realised that I had been advised not to eat takeaways during treatment. Actually, I only had a about a bite of it left. I finished it under the assumption that Burger King have stringent rules that their food is cooked to, and with a promise to myself not to forget in future. I might not have forgotten if I hadn't been so incredibly hungry.

Back home, I watched a bit of Jeremy Kyle (I know, but it's car crash TV and I can't help rubber necking.), then decided that today's guest was far too insane for my senses and turned over to watch Countdown. What? I am of that age, and I happen to like word games. However, I didn't get to the start of round two before deciding that I needed to sleep, so I switched off the TV, put my head against a cushion, and dropped straight off. When I woke up, 2 hours later, the dog was still on the other sofa, and I'm presuming she was snoring throughout my nap, and a neighbour's car was parked right outside my living room window. The car in question is a Honda somethingorother, and has a very loud engine, or maybe that's the exhaust, one way or another, it is usually possible to hear it coming from the moment it enters town, and I didn't even hear it park up right outside. This is a new form of sleeping; this is the kind of sleeping that babies do in the middle of a party. And I am only on week two of treatment.

I felt queasy when I woke up, like the morning after a good night out when some fool mentions fried eggs as a logical form of sustenance. Something was frying in the kitchen, something that I wanted to take outside and dump in the bin. Tom was cooking tea, steak and onions, but instead of the aroma being a mouth-watering temptation, it was a putrid stench that made me feel physically sick. The smell didn't just invade my nostrils; it seeped into my pores and threatened to overwhelm me. Remembering the anti sickness pills, I went into the dining room and took one, which put me in close contact with the offending food that I would normally enjoy. The tablet didn't stay down long, and for the first time since starting the treatment I had to run to the bathroom to be sick. So I then took another tablet, just to be on the safe side.

I could have gone to bed and curled up in self sympathy there and then, but I know that I have to keep a semblance of normality going, and so I went back into the living room and watched Emmerdale. However, by 7.30 I had enough, and decided that it was time to go to bed. I set the soaps to record, hoping that I would feel well enough to watch them at a later date, and carted myself upstairs for what turned out to be a better night's sleep than I have had since the PEG was first fitted. I can't say I slept all night without any disturbance, in fact I believe I woke up every 2 hours or so, but each time I woke I just looked at the time before putting my head back on the pillow and drifting off again, until 5.00 am, when I knew I had to get up. I don't know what time the driver is coming for me today, but my appointment is for 8.30, so

I had to make sure I was ready in time. Still my tummy is not quite right, and I couldn't face coffee when I got up, so instead I have had 2 cuppa soups.

My driver is here... have to go.

And home again with a day of chemotherapy and radiotherapy behind me once more. I nearly ran into the chemotherapy room when my name was called, I needed those anti sickness drugs so badly. If this is how it feels on week two, I dread to think what it is going to be like as the weeks go on.

Alison, the nurse who administered the drugs last week was doing the same job again. I had a question for her; the tingling, slightly stinging feeling that I get in my bum and nether regions when the anti sickness drug is put through my veins; do men...

'No, as far as I know they don't get it in their willy.' Alison giggled. 'Or if they do, they don't tell us about it.' She laughed.

Once again Val and Eddie were there in unison. Val made sure Eddie was settled in a chair next to me before going off to get him a bacon buttie from the shops across the road. I marvelled that he could still chomp into a bacon buttie as by this stage my mouth was sore, and the salt from the bacon would have been a bit too much for me to deal with.

I had noticed that Eddie and Val seemed a lot more familiar with the chemotherapy department than I was myself. They knew more of the nurses by their first names, and I wondered if this was because they lived more local than I did, so I asked, and found out that while Eddie had started the same treatment as myself at the same time I had started, and that we would be going through the same journey this time, Eddie was no stranger to the chemotherapy department.

I had assumed that as Eddie was going through the same treatment as me that he also had the same problems, an occult (hidden) cancer. But this is not the case with Eddie. They know where his tumour is, but it has tangled itself around veins, sinew and nerves, and at the moment is inoperable. So Eddie has been through two courses of chemotherapy so far, in the hope that it would have shrunk the tumour enough for them to operate, but sadly this was not successful enough, so now he has to go through the same aggressive radiotherapy as myself so that they will be able to get it down to operable size.

But he remains positive, because the doctors treating him are positive about his situation. They are confident that this treatment will shrink the tumour down so that they will be able to remove it without causing too much trauma to the surrounding tissue.

An old lady was attached up to a chemotherapy drip/pump just after Eddie and me. Her name was Joan, and later she was brought over to sit beside Val. The nurse asked:

'Are you alright there Joan?'

'No, I'm half left,' she replied, and we were to discover that this answer had been in complete honesty when she started to tell us how she shouldn't be there, that they shouldn't be giving her the treatment, and how she needed to get home for midday because her meal on wheels was being delivered then. Bless her, she was in a bit of a panic about missing the meals on wheels people, but as her treatment had started, she had to see it through to the end. It was gone midday when she left, but Sonia made sure she would have something to eat when she got home; a tuna and mayonnaise sandwich tucked into her bag.

While she was waiting to be unhooked from the drip, Joan told Val and I about how she had been mugged a year earlier; her bag had been snatched as she made her way to the shops and the only thing she got back was her bus pass that was found in the gutter later. Joan is in her 80s, she walks stooped and slowly, and how anyone could take advantage of this little old lady, how anyone could possibly harm a hair on her head, shooting is too good for such scumbags… in my humble opinion.

On the way back from Preston that day, Tony, my driver presented me with a bag of pear drops. His daughter had brought them for him when she had come to visit at the bank holiday and when he gave me one, and I could actually taste it properly, so he gave me the whole bag.

Friday 8th May 2009

My sense of taste is diminishing at a rate of knots now. The only thing I can taste properly is tomato soup. Not only is my sense of taste starting to go, so too is my sense of texture and consistency becoming heightened. Ground beef feels like little boulders in my mouth, and creamed potatoes have a strange consistency, almost gritty in texture. I know this because I ate shepherd's pie this evening, and while I finished it, I can't say I enjoyed it. Little did I realise when I ate this meal that it was my own, personal last supper.

I felt a sense of achievement today, finishing my second week of treatment. Yes my tongue is a bit sore, my mouth and throat is so dry at night that it keeps waking me up through the night, and I can no longer taste food, but I have got through 2 weeks of the travelling and treatment, and I'm still here.

I suspect that my sense of achievement is somewhat misplaced, and that I may be better off waiting until I have completed week 6 before I start slapping myself on the back. I say I can no longer taste food, but realistically I can still taste tomato soup, and I can still get a good flavour from warmed milk, even if the cornflakes I poured it on were like slivers of wet cardboard. I reckon that so long as the food is going down, and that so long as the lack of flavour doesn't make me feel sick, the important thing is that I am eating, that I am getting sustenance into my system. That said, I have been in touch with the nutritionists at Preston hospital to enquire about getting some food to put into the tube. I envisage the total lack of taste, when it finally descends, will put me off trying to eat in the normal sense. Besides, if the soreness in my mouth is anything to go by after only 2 weeks, there is no doubt I will need to use the feeding tube eventually.

The feeding tube: it has been sixteen days since it was inserted, and still my body is trying desperately to reject it. I find I have to clean away green gunge from the wound site several times a day, and the course of antibiotics given to me by my doctor hasn't totally cleared up the infection. It's still a tad sore, but it's not stopping me from sleeping any more, unless I turn over onto it, and I no longer feel a need to consume copious amounts of painkillers to deal with it.

In fact, the only painkillers I am using at the moment is an oral suspension of Paracetamol for the pain in my tongue. I'm not being a martyr, martyrdom is not my style, and I will take painkillers as and when I need them. I'm just not going to do so when it's not totally necessary.

Sunday 10th May 2009

I keep forgetting that even on days off from treatment the radiotherapy is still carrying on working in my system. I was reminded of this when I got up this morning to find my mouth in a worse state than ever. During the night I find that I keep waking up with a dry mouth; totally dry so that I have to keep a drink next to my bed. And over the past week or so I have got up to find my tongue coated in a white, viscous substance that I can only assume to be concentrated saliva. But this morning it was so much more than a thick white coating on my tongue; this morning it was more like a yellow blanket.

I tried to clear this with mouthwash, but after three attempts the yucky stuff was still clinging on in places, so I decided to get out the toothbrush and to gently try to clear it away with kiddie's toothpaste (bought in preparation for the treatment). Very gently, not wanting to cause any more pain than was already going on in my mouth, I brushed my tongue to clear the yellow gunge away, and immediately caused my tongue to start to bleed. The pain intensified somewhat, so my next step was to swallow some oral dihydrocodeine and to back this up with some Paracetamol suspension that again I hoped would stick to my mouth and provide palliative relief.

Actually, I'm quite proud of how I'm dealing with the pain so far. Oh I know, pride will probably come before a fall, and I will, over the coming weeks, learn that what I am suffering now isn't even close to real pain. But for now, two weeks and two days into my treatment, I am coping.

Melissa and Jade came to visit last night. I'm far too paranoid to get close to either of them for fear that they have been in contact with anyone suffering from swine flu, beriberi or the Ebola virus, but it was still good to see them both. I'm feeling somewhat isolated from society at the moment, although that is mostly by choice. I'm just so worried about picking up something that may set back my treatment. I read on the Macmillan website about a poor guy whose wife and children got a 24 hour bug that put him in hospital for 10 days. Surely, paranoia aside, it really has to be best to avoid any sort of contamination while this treatment is ongoing.

Melissa was eating a Mars Bar when she arrived, and while I wouldn't be able to eat any of it because my mouth is too sore, I held it under my nose and sniffed it at length.

Practical tip -

Do not eat a whole tin of baked beans while suffering from constipation as a result of taking painkillers; in particular not if you have a feeding tube fitted.

At last, a practical tip I can pass on to the reader. Last night I decided that I could eat a tin of baked beans. Coated in tomato sauce as they are, I knew I would be able to taste them. The texture was downright weird, not at all what I know baked beans to feel like in the mouth; they were like huge boulders, and although they were well cooked and quite soft, to me they were like little rocks. But I got them down, albeit slowly.

Oh but did I suffer for this during the night? Oh but am I still suffering for it now?

During the night I had dreadful wind that built up just under the site of the PEG fitment to the extent that I worried it was going to push it out. This morning I need to poo like never before, but absolutely nothing is happening other than a strange groaning noise from my tummy. All I can do is take the Movicol and wait for something to happen, which it will eventually; I just have to be a patient patient once again.

So… don't eat too many beans… you have been warned!

Monday 11th May 2009

Things started changing again yesterday. I noticed mid afternoon that I had developed a rash, similar to prickly heat, around my neck that dissipated around the top of my boobs. It's itchy, and rather unsightly, and I must mention it when I get to Preston today.

Tom made some homemade tomato soup with basil yesterday. I managed to get that down and still taste it, although not as strongly as homemade soup would usually taste. Later on I had a can of Ambrosia creamed rice, with some seedless raspberry jam stirred into it. I could hardly taste this at all, but I got it down anyway, seeing as my throat is not actually too sore to eat as yet. Later again I had a mug of Bovril, which I may have made a bit too strong as I could definitely taste the salt in it. But in general, my taste buds are not working as well as they should be; not even *close* to what they should be.

I have turned into a bit of a food tourist and find myself making a small whimpering noise at the sight of a small boy dipping soldiers into a soft boiled egg on a TV advert. I watched several hours of Come Dine With Me, revelling in the sights of the food that I could neither smell nor taste.

I watched Desperate Housewives, and the parts that stand out in my memory are the scenes containing food; oatmeal, macaroons, ice-cream… I could taste them all in my head, but I knew my senses would not be likely to cooperate with the real thing.

And still the wind built up in my tummy. All of yesterday evening my stomach groaned and creaked, desperate for some sort of relief from the constipation and wind that comes as a side effect of the drugs. And while the last thing I needed was to add to this feeling of being as bloated as a basking seal, I knew I was going to have to take some painkillers if I was going to get a decent night's sleep.

My tongue is sore, and over the past couple of nights I have woken time and time again because of the dryness inside my mouth. I needed to sleep properly, without the soreness and dryness waking me every couple of hours, and so I took dihydrocodeine and Paracetamol, both in liquid form, before applying liberal amounts of cream to my neck and face and getting off to bed.

It worked… I slept like the proverbial baby, only waking every 5 hours or so; not for a feed but for a top-up of the drugs that allowed me to get a half way decent night's sleep, interspersed with strange dreams. I dreamed I owned a snow covered shopping mall. When I say snow covered, I mean it was covered in snow on the inside. The shoe shop in the mall sold the most beautiful shoes for little girls, but the strange people who lived on the other side of town, who spoke in whistles and bleeps, were not allowed inside my shopping mall, and they were certainly not allowed any of the pretty shoes for their children.

Then this morning arrived at 6.55 am, along with a rather bad sore throat. Rather bad? I don't know about the 'scale of 1 – 10' thing. Surely that scale has to be subjective at every point. As I have already stated, I would not consider myself to have a pain threshold at all, and yet here I am at 7.30 in the morning, sitting in front of the laptop writing about how the pain is before I actually go and take something for it, so can it really be that bad?

I'm not being a martyr; I just wanted to write about how I feel before I get rid of the feeling, if that makes sense. And as the pain is really only there when I swallow, so long as I refrain from swallowing too much, it's bearable I suppose. OK, if pushed I would say the pain is at a 1 while not swallowing and goes up to about a 3 while swallowing.

Now you see; if most people wrote about their experiences as I am doing I am sure that a 3 would not even be worth a mention. But 3 got me out of bed and downstairs; 3 is a figure I considered worthy of literary recognition; 3 refused to allow me any further sleep. Which just shows what a dreadful wimp I really am.

Yet, conversely, I am coping well enough with 3 that I haven't yet taken any painkillers. Even though a little fear is niggling at the back of my mind, asking me how the hell I am going to cope when the pain reaches 10, at the moment I am coping with the pain, and even if I do only class it as a 3, I'm not crying, I'm not feeling sorry for myself, I'm still at a stage where I am simply getting on with it.

Then again, it is only the start of week 3. Hmmm, the number 3 seems to be significant today.

It is now 8.00 am, the sun is shining, the sky is blue, and I should be heading off to the station to get the train to go to work. But instead I am about to go to the bathroom to flush through my feeding tube before getting ready for the day ahead. And I can tell you, I would much rather be going to work.

Tuesday 12th May 2009

I was horribly sick yesterday evening. I had made it as far as the bathroom, but to neither the sink nor the toilet before I vomited all over the floor. I hate to be sick, and will fight it to the last, but yesterday evening there was nothing I could to about it. It was violent, projectile and it tore at my throat. Tom simply took me into the living room, then went and cleaned it up. Hero!

Today I had to be up at 5.00 am to make sure I am ready in time to leave at 6 if necessary. I think I had a pretty bad night, but as I am only on week three of the treatment I probably don't know what a bad night is yet. I went to bed at 8 last night, after taking plenty of painkillers to make sure that the soreness in my mouth didn't keep me awake. I awoke again at around midnight, my throat sore again, and so took more painkillers. I am ever wary of how long it has been since I last took some; the last thing I need to do is to overdose, although I can fully see why anyone in constant pain could accidentally take too much medication. I woke up every couple of hours or so after this, but only took Paracetamol at about 3 am. The rash is still rather itchy, and I had to splash cold water on my skin during the night to try to cool it down a bit.

For some years now I have been looking in the mirror in the morning and wondering who that middle-aged woman was that looked back at me. As with most people, I still expect to see the girl I once was in the mirror, and it is ever a shock to see that she will never come back.

But today was different. Today I didn't see a middle aged woman in the mirror. Today I saw a child, a frightened child, a wide-eyed child who didn't seem to understand what was going on in her life.

Saturday 16th May 2009

When I started to write this I made a promise to myself that I would do my best to write every day, if only a few words. But now it seems that I cannot keep that promise to myself. I haven't written a word since Tuesday morning, mainly because I have simply been too busy with medications and the tube in the mornings and too tired by the time I get home from Preston in the afternoons.

Tuesday at chemo was trying. The nurse who tried to get a line into the back of my right hand failed twice when the vein 'blew'. I'm not sure what it means for a vein to 'blow' but it doesn't sound too nice and it has left a huge, black bruise on the back of my hand. It didn't particularly hurt, the vein just refused to have anything to do with the needle that nurse was trying to insert. So over to the left hand, and the needle went in straight away. I have the kind of veins a junkie would kill for, so I pity anyone with poor veins going through chemotherapy. Apparently it is the chemo that makes veins difficult to get to.

Eddie and Val were already there by the time I got my line in, and Eddie appeared to be in good form, even though he said he was getting a bit of a sore throat and food wasn't tasting the same. However, when Val went out to the shops for his papers she also left on a hunt for a meat and potato pie, which Eddie ate with gusto on her return. She asked if I wanted anything; '…a packet of wine gums please'. That was all I could stomach in the way of food.

By Tuesday I had realised that I was going to have to start tube feeding. And in spite of the horrors I went through actually having the damn thing fitted, I am, as Dr Siva said I would be, grateful for it now. While I can still smell food, I can't taste even tomato soup now, and when I tried to do so yesterday it tasted so gross and it burned my throat. Even water is bad, and is more like baby oil than a refreshing drink. So, after much consultation with dieticians, doctors and chemist shops, I am now pouring high protein, high vitamin drinks down my tube several times a day.

However, when they calculated what my normal daily calorific content would be they only asked what I had for breakfast, lunch and dinner, they didn't ask how many Kit-Kats, Revels, crisps and bottles of wine I may consume in a week. So this was left out of the sums when it came to deciding how many bottles of supplement food I would need each day. Hence, in the first week I have already lost half a stone in weight.

Food has become an obsession. I was watching TV last night when someone took a packet of processed ham out of a fridge. You know the stuff, shiny, pink, swimming in water, and the kind of food I would usually turn my nose up at in favour of my butcher's ham that he cooks on the premises. But last night I wanted that whole packet of ham. Not only did I want that whole packet of ham, I also wanted a box of Dairylea triangles to go with it. Every advert for food on TV makes me sigh inwardly, and sometimes audibly. At the moment I feel like an inactive bulimic. If I could taste food I could happily sit in front of the fridge stuffing my face before throwing it all back up just so that I could start all over again.

It's not a hunger thing; the food supplements seem to cover the hunger side of my dietary needs. It's a need to taste food in a way that I have never experienced in my life. You know that feeling when you have had to much to drink and all you want is a hot dog or a kebab that you wouldn't normally touch with a bargepole, and it's like your life depends on it, it's like that is the best food you have ever had in your life. Well, for me this feeling is that, intensified a hundredfold.

On Tuesday, after chemo, we picked up another guy who was heading our way after his appointment at Preston. Oh, I was so tired; all I wanted was to sit there quietly, watching the fields and traffic go past, until I could get home and relax. But the guy that we picked up talked incessantly all the way to his front door. When I say incessantly, I mean he just never bloody well shut up, not for longer than four seconds, I know because I counted. He spoke in a monotone, northern drone about fish, his holidays, fish, his holidays, fish… until I wanted to slap him across the back of the head with a large fish and tell him to shut the fuck up! For a full hour and a half he talked about himself, and I am sure he could have continued to do so if we had carried on to Aberdeen and beyond. In fact, I wonder if he talks in his sleep.

As the week has gone on my symptoms from the treatment have continued to escalate, but I am still here, still getting up every morning to wait for the car to take me to hospital, and now that three weeks are out of the way, I am half way through the treatment. Although, as I am sure anyone who has been through this would agree, it is more like torture than treatment.

Apart from not being able to eat because of the way food tastes so disgusting, I am also suffering with sleep problems because of the dry mouth and sore throat. I am going through bottles and bottles of mouthwash in an attempt to clear my tongue and throat of the sticky residue that is all my saliva is by now. As I write now I am trying to drink a cup of warm, strong tea. Surprisingly I can taste it a little, so I may continue to drink more throughout the day, as dehydration is another thing that concerns me. Whenever I think of it I go and pour water down the tube just to make sure that my body doesn't start to dry out.

So, on a scale of 1 – 10... just how bad is it now?

It's hard to judge really. I mean, I'm now sitting here writing this, so I'm not bedridden, I'm not rolling around in agony or anything like that. My mouth is clogged up with thick saliva, my throat hurts when I swallow, I want food like I can't tell you, but in general I do believe I am coping so far. And if *I* can cope, I believe anyone can.

I'm not saying it's easy, not by a long way. In fact, some days I can get so down that I feel like bursting into tears. But again, on the plus side, this is something I have not actually done, not yet anyway, not since my experience with Mr Mian.

I have had to put a notice in my front door that reads 'NO COLD CALLERS PLEASE' owing to the fact that it seems as though every afternoon there is another knock on the door to disturb me just as I am trying to have a rest. Double glazing salespeople, who seem incapable of noticing that my windows are practically brand new; charity collectors, whom I do not want to have to explain to that I already give to charities I chose myself; politicians, like I give a shit which one of them gets an expense account at the elections in June.

Near the start of this book I berated the politicians and their expense accounts that siphon money from the taxpayer while charities such as cancer research have to beg the public for funds. But this week the expenses scandal has come to a head in a way that the British public never anticipated.

I think it is now safe to say that I was not exaggerating when I said that politicians are creaming the expense sheets in order to live in the kind of opulence that the ordinary man on the street can only dream of. It turns out that not only are we paying for second homes for these people, we are also paying for massage chairs, plasma TVs, and all sorts of luxury items that the average tax payer has to fork out for from their own pockets.

Yesterday, David Cameron abandoned his planned party political broadcast to instead try to allay the fears of the British voters that his people would not be claiming any such expenses for personal items. But he left me shaking my head with his assurances that his people would only claim for legitimate expenses; the likes of council tax, utility bills and interest on mortgages.

Excuse me!

My wage doesn't come close to comparing with that of a politician, but I pay my own council tax, utility bills and my own bloody mortgage. I cannot even begin to understand how Mr Cameron, or anyone else, can justify such bills being paid by the taxpayer when they are in receipt of enormous salaries to start with.

Ok, so they have to move to London to do their jobs; well so do a lot of other people, and they don't get their bills paid for them. A good friend of mine moved to London to be a Policewoman, a vital job that doesn't pay anything like a politician's salary, but she has to pay her own bills.

This week I also met Beryl (not her real name). Beryl is in her 80s and lives in sheltered accommodation with her husband, also in his 80s and severely disabled. Beryl's husband needs a lot of personal care because of his disability, and when it was found that Beryl needed chemotherapy and radiotherapy in order to kill off the cancer in her bowel, they had to make the heart rending decision that her husband go into a care home while she is having her treatment. Like myself she is away from home for anything up to 7 hours a day, and as her husband cannot be left on his own for this long, they really had no other choice. I know that Beryl is counting the days until she can have her beloved husband home again.

Beryl's husband's care is costing them almost £500 per week, a cost that they have to foot themselves because there is nowhere else for them to turn for help. Obviously they can afford to pay it; otherwise Beryl's husband would not be in the care home in the first place.

But they are not wealthy people. If they were wealthy people they would not be living in sheltered housing. What little savings they have is being eaten up because they have to pay for a 'second home' for Beryl's husband while she receives her treatment. There are no expense accounts for Beryl and her husband to claim on, they cannot plunder the tax coffers that they paid into for many years so that her husband's care bill can be subsidised while she receives her life saving treatment.

Yet Shahid Malik, the Justice Minister, can claim for a massage chair because he has a bad back, and David Chaytor has claimed £13,000 in mortgage interest for a property with no outstanding mortgage.

This is not a simple case of people doctoring their expense sheets to get a little extra mileage on their cars, or a meal on the company. This is blatant theft, this is obtaining money by deception, and I only hope that all of those involved in the scandal will be punished as the criminals they are.

This cannot be looked on as 'whoops, did I tick the wrong box?' These people knew exactly what they were doing when they put in claims for their luxuries, and their living expenses, and it really is about time that politicians start to pay their own bills and stop being leeches on society. Earlier I said they were like some sort of benefits cheats, but really, their audacious use of the system goes far beyond that. The politicians who clam expenses where they are not allowed to are little more than fraudsters, and should be dealt with as such.

Will I be voting in the next elections? Will I shite! Really, what is the point? They say what they think you want to hear, then they just go and do their own thing anyway.

Politicians are in it for themselves, for the money, for the political clout, for the expenses and for the kudos they crave.

And Beryl, like the rest of us, she will struggle on and pay her bills herself.

Monday 18th May 2009

And another weekend has passed. I have managed to get through a whole two days without giving up. Not that giving up is anything close to an option right now.

The morning continued on a downward spiral when I threw up the food supplements a few minutes after pouring them down the tube and into my tummy. I hate the taste of bananas, but I had used a banana flavoured Ensure drink because I can't taste what is going down the tube. But unfortunately I can taste things on the way back up. It was a bad start to the day, and things only continued to get worse as the day went on.

My driver turned up to collect me, and could see by my face that I wasn't feeling too good. My stomach was sick, my throat was sore, and the 70 mile journey was undertaken in almost complete silence. I didn't want to talk to anyone, about anything. I just wanted to go to sleep, but that's not possible in a moving car.

It seemed to take forever to get to Preston; as we pulled up outside the cancer unit, the cancer unit with numerous signs declaring the area to be a non-smoking area, there was a man standing there smoking.

Ooooh this gets me mad. I don't know whether he was a patient or a carer, or a driver, all I know is that when I get to the radiotherapy unit I do not want to walk through a haze of smoke to get into the building. Giving up smoking was very hard for me, and took me over two years in total. And now that I have managed to stop completely I find it wholly insulting that some people don't have enough grace, decency, common sense and respect for cancer patients that they cannot take their 'cancer sticks' off around the corner.

'Hello!' I said to the man, too enraged to even *try* to hide my disgust. 'Can't you read? Or don't you understand the pictures?' I said to him, pointing at the no smoking signs that didn't really need any words to deliver their clear message. Wordlessly, he put out his cigarette on the ground, and I flounced off into the building, my anger giving me a little energy if nothing else.

Perhaps it is condesending of me to feel this way about smoking, after all I was a 40 a day woman until 2 years ago, when I managed to cut it down to 2 a day, until diagnosed with cancer again this year, which has made me stop smoking for good. Oh I hope it has made me stop smoking for good. I don't want to tempt fate in any way, but I never want to smoke again. I never want to smell like that again. I cannot believe how bad the smell is from people who smoke and I am embarrassed to think that I went around stinking like that; like an old ashtray in an old pub that hasn't been washed out properly since Walter Raleigh first brought tobacco back from the Americas. If smokers realised how bad the smell is I am sure it would encourage more people to stop smoking. Surely nobody wants to go around smelling like that.

The man outside the cancer unit that day is not the only one I have seen smoking there. While there are not many people so uncaring as to smoke around the building, there are some who really don't seem to care so long as they get to drag smoke into their lungs. There is one woman in particular that I have seen smoking around the building on many occasions. She is a young woman, obviously having treatment as she is bald and wears a bandana; so this indicates she is suffering from cancer, somewhere within her body, and yet she takes any available opportunity to pump more poison into her system while the doctors are trying to cure her. I was walking down the corridor from the main hospital to the radiotherapy unit one day when the stench of smoke hit me; a little farther along the corridor there was an open doorway, and this young woman was just outside the doorway, sucking frantically on the cigarette she needed so badly that this was the furthest away she could get; not giving a damn that the fumes were drifting down the corridor for everyone else to breathe in.

Another day a man was called in for his treatment, and his elderly wife told the radiologist that her husband had gone outside for a cigarette. If this wasn't bad enough, when the man in question came back into the waiting room he was being wheeled in a wheelchair because he only had one leg!

So, the bad day didn't get much better as the waiting time for the machine was 30 minutes. Usually I didn't mind waiting, but on Monday I just wanted to get it over with and get home. Eventually it was my turn, the mask was fitted in place and clipped to the radiology table, and the treatment carried on, buzzing and whirring around my head.

It seemed to take forever to get home that day; an hour and a half can seem like an eternity when all you want is the comfort of your own home. Once home I took some anti-sickness medication, but still felt really rough. That said, I managed to sleep for an hour and a half before waking up feeling even more sick. I made it to the bathroom, but not to a receptacle in which to deposit the contents of my stomach. In a scene reminiscent of The Exorcist I threw up all over the bathroom floor once again, what looked like metal filings in vomit. It was projectile vomiting at its worst, and it refused to stop.

When the violent reaction my body was having to the treatment finally subsided I went and got the mop bucket from under the stairs, which was taken out of my hands by Tom who arrived at that very moment and sent me into the living room while he cleaned up my mess for me again. What a hero.

Tuesday 19th May 2009

I now hate Tuesdays with a passion. I have to be up at 5.00 am every Tuesday morning to make sure that I have time to get ready before my driver arrives. I find that I no longer have time to write on a morning, other than to make the occasional note, and that my time is taken up by other necessities. First I have to try to clear my mouth of the gunge that has built up over the night. I gargle with mouthwash, then wash my mouth out again, but still the yellow mucus sticks like glue to my tongue. Then I have to take some of my medication, my anti sickness drugs, before I can start to feed myself via the tube. On Tuesday morning I made sure I took the anti-sickness drugs before feeding because I was in dread of throwing up again like I had done twice on the Monday. However, in spite of this, almost as soon as the food was in my stomach it was propelled back up at an alarming rate, and I couldn't face trying to force myself to pour more food down the tube, just in case it came back up again.

My driver turned up at 7.00 am, and the journey to Preston was again undertaken in almost complete silence. I was afraid to talk in case I vomited; and besides, I had nothing to talk about, apart from how horribly sick I felt. All I wanted was to be at the hospital, and to have the wonderful anti sickness medicine pumped into my veins so that this dreadful sick feeling would go away.

Normally I have very good veins, and have never had trouble getting needles inserted in the back of my hands or in my arms. But now I was beginning to have problems. The week before two veins had burst while the nurse tried to put the cannula into the back of my hand, and this time my veins were trying to hide altogether. I had to stand with my hands in a sink filled with hot water in an attempt to encourage my veins to stand out a little. It took a few minutes, but it worked.

Eddie and Val were there as usual, but Eddie was in pain. I had seen them both the day before at the radiotherapy unit, and Eddie was in dreadful pain with his back, both sides, and he was worried that it was his kidneys. We agreed on our level of overall suffering, and that we seemed to be getting to the same place at the same time with regards to the effects of the treatment, but I could see that Val was beside herself with worry over this new pain that was keeping Eddie awake at night.

The chairs in the oncology unit are recliners, and so I reclined the chair, put a pillow behind my head, and tried to relax as best I could. I felt exhausted, a new level of tiredness had set in, and all I really wanted to do was to sleep. But because I was one of those babies that was tiptoed around by over-zealous parents, I have never been able to sleep unless I have total silence, and preferably darkness. Which is why I wear earplugs at night and have heavy curtains at my bedroom window. I couldn't sleep, but I could relax, there was nothing for me to do other than read a bit, and wait for the poisons to flow through my system and kill off the cancer cells that were hiding somewhere.

I had asked to see a doctor in order to ask for some stronger painkillers. I don't know if I'm just being a dreadful wimp, but the dihydrocodeine just doesn't seem to be working as well as it had been. Not only that, it stung like mad when I swallowed it, so I decided to ask the doctor for oromorph, the morphine that they supply to patients going through this treatment.

I was a bit scared of the idea of taking morphine, worried that it may become an addiction, even though the doctors assured me this would not happen. Most of the time my throat is not sore, but when I try to swallow… oh boy, that's when the measure of how bad the pain can be really shows itself. The doctor I spoke to at the hospital agreed to give me the morphine, and told me that I should try one 5ml dose, and if that wasn't enough I could double that. And when I got home that's exactly what I did. He had already told me that one 5ml dose was the equivalent to codeine, and as dihydrocodeine was not cutting the mustard, I didn't see much point in taking something that would have a lesser effect so I went straight on to two 5ml spoonfuls.

On the first day of my chemotherapy treatment, when I had met Ann, she had told me about a book she had read by a cancer sufferer, but I had completely forgotten that she has said she would leave it at the unit for me. A nurse came over and gave me the book, by Jill Ireland, Charles Bronson's wife, it chronicled her first encounter with cancer.

But not only was Jill's story different from mine in that her cancer was in her breast, it was also a world away from my experience in that she, a wealthy celebrity, the wife of a famous movie star, followed a different path in her quest for a cure.

Jill's doctor called round to her house to see her; Jill's room at the hospital was private; Jill tried any whacky, wayout 'cures' that she came into contact with; Jill didn't need to organise free transport, she just chose a car from the garage… a collection that included a Rolls Royce.

I read Jill Ireland's book from cover to cover, but the only things I found we had in common was our inability to prevent vomiting. It was as I read this book that I realised how the celebrity, the wealthy and the influential people of this world go through a completely different experience to the lesser mortals, such as myself, Eddie, and the many wonderful people I have met on my journey.

Recently, Max Clifford told how he had paid Jade Goody's medical bills when the NHS failed her. He didn't elaborate on this statement, and I am still at a loss to understand how the NHS failed Jade. Did they refuse to treat her? I can't imagine so. Did they refuse to give her a private room unless she paid? Perhaps. I really don't know how they 'failed' her, because they have certainly never failed me.

I don't think I would like the isolation and loneliness of private medical treatment. OK, the treatment rooms may be posher, the upholstery may be plusher, but I would truly hate to be stuck on my own in a private room; much preferring the company of other people. Jill Ireland was surrounded by people prepared to take her money for all sorts of alternative treatments; did she really believe these money grabbers cared whether or not she survived?

One therapist taught her to meditate, yes, that's a cure for cancer.

Another gave her bottles of electrically charged water to drink and 'shot' electromagnetic charges through her body, for a huge fee of course.

It seemed to me while reading her book that there was only one person she needed to be there for her, and that was her husband, Charles Bronson. But if he was there for her, it was not in the complete way that Tom is there for me, nor in the dedicated way that Val is there for Eddie.

Two weeks after a mastectomy, Jill was having sex with her husband. Shocked? I was. She was in dreadful pain, her wounds were not close to healing, and I am sure no woman who was going through the pain and suffering that Jill Ireland was wanted to have sex at that point. But what beggars belief more than anything is that, even if she were feeling so horny that she was begging for sex, her husband didn't have the decency to back off, to protect her from the possibility of being hurt. Jill told it in a way that said she laid her head on his shoulder and things developed until they were making love… yet it came across as though she were desperately trying to hold on to her man, that her fear of him rejecting her because of the disease is what drove her to please him, and not just with sex.

Charles needed to go to Vermont on holiday, so she encouraged him to go, right in the middle of her treatment. I can't imagine Tom leaving me for a day, let alone weeks on end while I am going through this treatment. And I know that Val would rather cut her own head off than leave Eddie to go through his treatment alone.

Then there was the night they were getting ready to go out to dinner and Jill suddenly needed to tell her husband how she felt, how scared she was… and, instead of taking her in his arms and comforting her, he got annoyed and told her that her timing was misplaced.

Jill Ireland put her care into the hands of quacks and therapists, she spoke to strangers on the phone about what she was going through, she relied on her friend Alan to help her through the dark times, because her husband seemed to be incapable of finding the strength necessary to support his wife through the bad days. Sometimes he told her he would go through it for her if he could; but they are just words. When Tom tells me that he would gladly take the disease and treatment from me, that he would rather it were him suffering… he backs it up with all he does. When Charles Bronson told his wife he would go through it for her if he could, he backed his words up by going off on a skiing holiday and leaving her to cope alone.

For anyone to say that the NHS does not provide the very best of treatment to cancer sufferers is an insult to the dedicated doctors, nurses and radiographers who devote their time and care to their patients. Never once have I felt like a number, there has not been any occasion when I felt that I could have received better care from Preston hospital if it had all been pre-arranged by BUPA. My care givers are wonderful people. OK, they may not remember me next year, but that will not be because they don't care, or because I am not famous, it will be because they will be dedicating their care to those who need it at the time.

Saturday 23rd May 2009

Oh the luxury of a weekend off from the travelling. I am going to slob out for the day, stay in my pyjamas, watch TV and do absolutely nothing. I had a bad night's sleep again last night. The dry mouth thing is really disturbing my sleep badly. Every hour or so I am waking up with my mouth totally dry and if I try to swallow (nothing) it hurts like hell. Dr Siva prescribed a spray of artificial saliva for me the other day, and I now keep this by my bed at night, but it doesn't last all that long, and so I keep waking and have to use it over and over during the night. I can't help worrying that this is going to disturb my sleep in the future, when I need a full night's sleep to be ready for work the next morning.

I can't wait to get back to work. At the moment I am aiming at being back in the office by October; I don't think that's being too optimistic. But I worry that my disturbed sleep will make it difficult, and I worry that the dry mouth will make it difficult to talk on the phone all day. But I shouldn't be worrying, worry never made anything any easier in this life.

The hunger is starting to drive me nuts. I am longing for certain foods. More than anything I want a bowl of Chili con Connolly (made with baked beans rather than kidney beans) with a pile of hot buttered toast, with the butter dripping from the toast. Surprisingly, I'm not bothered about chocolate, something I really thought I would lust after. I imagine that eating chocolate is going to be rather difficult once the treatment is complete. If I am left with a dry mouth as a permanent thing, then it will be very hard to eat chocolate.

I was talking to my granddaughter Jade online this morning. I've given up on trying to talk to people on the phone because the mouth mucus and because, the dryness makes it very difficult to hold conversations. We made a couple of plans for when I am better. We are going to go horse riding together. We are both terrified of horses, wary of heights, and rather nervous about the idea, but it's still something we want to do, so we are planning to overcome our fears together.

Next year sometime we intend on going to London, just the two of us, to take in all the palaces and the Tower of London. We have a mutual interest in history, particularly the Tudor period, that nobody else in our family shares, so we are going to take the trip together. Jade loves history, so it will be good for her to see the actual places where Elizabeth I and her contemporaries lived.

Another plan, although somewhat adventurous, is a trip to New York. At the moment I'm not sure when we may be able to afford it but it would be so good. I want to ride in a yellow cab and Jade wants to shop at Bloomingdales. Ah, we can but dream. Whether or not I will be up for the long haul flight, even if I do get the money together, well, that remains to be seen, but for now there's no harm in hoping.

Sunday 24th May 2009

'The night went by slowly… like the great black wheels of a juggernaut.'

Words within a book by Graham Masterton, a book that I read many years ago, the title of which evades my recollection right now, but words that I remembered nonetheless, because I hadn't got the foggiest idea what he meant by those words at the time.

The book in question is about a restaurant critic working in the Cajun area of the deep south of the US. The 'hero' of the book discovers that a secret restaurant is serving up bits and pieces of its willing members, in order to ultimately end up with one person who has consumed everyone else. And one night of vigil went by '… like the great black wheels of a juggernaut.'

I have read many, many books over the years, usually I have at least 2 on the go at the same time, but it is rare that I recall lines from books as readily as I did that one when I woke up this morning. And now I think I know what he meant.

You know when you're on the motorway in a car, and to take the next exit you have to start undertaking other vehicles, and then all of a sudden there's a great big truck on your right hand side that could crush you in a second, should the driver lose one second's concentration. The great black wheels seem to go by so slowly, so menacingly that when you get past it your mind breathes a huge sigh of relief that you are not going to end up as mincemeat. That's what Graham Masterton meant when he said the night went by slowly, like the great black wheels of a juggernaut.

What am I waffling on about?

That's what last night was for me, a long, painful night that seemed to go on forever.

I decided not to take the morpine before I went to bed last night. I seem to have gone through what I was given last Tuesday very quickly, and have less than half a bottle left. So instead I decided to take dihydrocodeine and paracetamol, really believing that it would be enough to get me through the night. But it wasn't. I woke up at 1.00 am unable to swallow with the pain, and had to come back downstairs to take some morphine after all.

However, I hadn't got my timing right, and had only left 2 hours between taking the dihydrocodeine and the morphine. While I'm not taking enough to kill myself accidentally, the combined effects of the drugs had a bad reaction within my brain, and although I fell asleep very quickly when I went back to bed, it was to have nightmare after nightmare, waking me again and again.

It's all well and good to say that they are only dreams, but at the time they are real, and even when we wake from nightmares we are left holding on to the emotions that we were feeling when asleep and in torment.

At one time I dreamed I was being held fast by an unseen, hairy creature in my bed. Held in a vice like grip I could not get free from the creature's hold nor from its disgusting stench. I fought, I struggled, I gouged at its body, but only wakefulness got me away from the monster that had been supplied, I assume, by the combined effects of the morphine and dihydrocodeine.

I won't do that again!

Another thing that is keeping me awake is that I cannot wear earplugs at the moment because my ears seem rather sensitive. I don't know if this is as a result of the radiotherapy, but whenever I try to put the earplugs in I get a stinging sensation that is not possible to relax with. So I am having to try to sleep without them, and next door's dogs are simply not co-operating. That said, neither are their owners, who live in a different time zone… somewhere in Russia I think.

I'm not entirely sure how many little dogs live next door, but I think it's somewhere around the count of 10. They are chiwowas and shitsues (yes, I am fully aware that both of those names are spelt wrong, but you get the gist, and I don't care) and their combined yapping could probably lift the roof from Fort Knox. Their owners are out for most of the day, so they bark at anything that moves. And when their owners come in at night, often after 10.00 pm, their barking takes on frantic proportions. Later, much later, the owners go to bed and the dogs bark on and off throughout the night. The owners don't get up until midday (early morning in some part of Russia) so they also bark incessantly throughout the morning.

So, without exaggeration, the dogs are barking almost constantly.

And I hear what you're saying 'Do something about it.'

And of course there are options. I could knock on their door and tell them that the dogs barking is driving me crazy. After all, they know that I am going through this treatment and I am sure they would be understanding. But what would they do about it? Would they get rid of their beloved dogs just because they are disturbing me while I am so exhausted? Probably, and if they did I couldn't live with myself. I can't imagine how much it would hurt if I had to get rid of Molly because a neighbour couldn't put up with her noise (not that Molly is noisy). I would rather move house first. Now there's a thought. If I were to tell them perhaps they would move house and take the dogs with them. But then that begs the question of who might move into the house if they moved out.

No, fuck it, I'll just have to put up with the yappy little bastards. Eventually I will be better and I won't hate them like I do now. I won't hate them like I did when I woke up this morning with my throat feeling like I had swallowed a razor blade and all I wanted to do was to go back to sleep but there really was not a chance of that happening.

The pain was so bad this morning that I could have cried if I was the crying type. Instead of crying I got out of bed, came downstairs, and started the morning ritual of oral hygeine, medication and feeding via the tube. And this morning there was no hesitation when it came to choosing pain relief; only morphine was going to touch this pain.

I don't think I'm going to do much for the rest of the day. I have to email friends to let them know how I'm getting on, as telephone conversations are out of the question while my throat is this sore. Then I suppose it is a day of TV while the rest of the country enjoys the sunshine of the bank holiday weekend.

Wednesday 1st July 2009

No, you haven't put your bookmarker in the wrong place or skipped a few pages by accident, it really is the first of July today and it has been several weeks since I have worked on this book in any way other than to make the occasional note.

Morning after morning the laptop stared at me accusingly but I ignored its best efforts to seduce me into writing. I simply could not do it, I was too tired, too sick and too drugged up. My mind became the prisoner of Morpheus. Not the character from the move The Matrix (I have never seen the movie), but the Greek God of dreams whom morphine is named in honour of. Maybe 'honour' is the wrong word to use there, as my mind was more enslaved than honoured.

As the treatment contiued, so too did the side effects escalate. But because the side effects gradually increased it was possible to take them on as and when they appeared, even if it was not possible for me to write about it.

Over the next couple of weeks my life took on a quality of sameness, while paradoxically changing every day. Morning ablutions now included taking breakfast through my tube, followed by taking increasing medication which could only be administered in the same way as soon it was not even possible to swallow the smallest amount of medication. Then it would be off to Preston, have the treatment, back from Preston, sleep for a few hours, watch TV for a while then off to bed again before repeating the entire process once more.

Sometimes I doubted that I would get to the end of the treatment, and the fifth of June seemed an eternity away. But somehow I did it; I got up every day, I got to Preston every day, and eventually the fifth of June came around.

Most days I hardly spoke to the driver, or to the other people who were in the car. The build up of mucus in my mouth got so bad that eventually I was taking several sheets of kitchen towel (ordinary tissues were not strong enough) with me to hospital, trying to spit the contents of my mouth into this as discreetly as possible. I have no idea where it was coming from, but for me it was a worse side effect than the pain. The pain could be controlled, but the mucus just kept coming, getting thicker every day.

When the day came for my final bout of chemotherapy I wished there were some other way of getting to the hospital, something like the teleporter from Star Trek would have been nice. I dreaded the journey; I felt so sick that I just wanted to crawl back into bed and go to sleep, but I felt too sick to sleep, and the only way I was going to get any relief was to get to the hospital and have the injection of medicine that would make me feel better.

The journey was horrendous, and seemed to take forever, but eventually the car stopped outside the oncology department of Preston hospital, and I stumbled out and made my way inside.

The receptionist was on the phone when I went up to the counter, so I waited. But my legs wouldn't hold me up properly, so I leaned forward to support myself on the counter. I felt as though I could collapse at any moment, and while it was probably only seconds, it seemed like an age before the receptionist realised I was in a bad way and told me to go straight through to the main room.

Even with the Ondansetron (anti sickness medication) in my veins, I still felt dreadful. I was exhausted, and so I reclined my chair and laid back with my feet up. Sonia was desperate to do something to help me, but there was nothing anyone could do, I just had to lay there and wait. After a few hours the drug did its work, and I started to feel a little better.

I had intended to get a big box of chocolates for the girls who worked on Linear Amplfier number 5, but I didn't. The intention was there, but the ability to go to the shop and purchase one was not. The build-up of mucus in my mouth made it very difficult to speak, and I would have found it very difficult to make a shopkeeper understand what it was that I wanted to purchase. What time I didn't spend at the hospital I spent sleeping, and I simply did not get around to buying the chocolates. I will get them, I will say thank you to the teams both at radiology and at chemotherapy, but for now I need to concentrate on getting well.

Although I had been warned that the radiation would continue to work inside my body for a couple of weeks after the treatment was complete, I had a misguided notion that it would be easier to bear because I would not have all the travelling to deal with. I was wrong! Once the treatment was finished the symptoms continued to escalate until by the end of the second week I felt so sick that I couldn't think straight. I couldn't bear the smell or sight of food, and there were no warnings as to when I would be physically sick.

The skin on my neck had been red and sore; so much so that I was getting up several times a night to put on more cream. But by the end of the fortnight after completion of treatment the skin on my neck was no longer red, it was purple and in some places it had split and cracked and was bleeding.

But there was no going back. The treatment had finished, so it wasn't possible for me to say: OK, I've had enough, I want to stop now. That simply was not an option any more. All I could do was suffer the consequences, keep taking the drugs, and wait for things to improve.

I was supposed to be going to hospital on the Thursday following the completion of the treatment, but even though I had managed to get ready for the journey, I realised, about half an hour before my transport was due to arrive, that there was no way I could make the journey to Preston. I felt so sick that I was sure I would not get out of town before needing to throw up. So I cancelled the appointment, even though it was short notice, and it was another week before I could make it to Preston.

The pain aspect has not really bothered me too much over the past few weeks. Taking so much morphine, topped up by voltarol, paracetamol and every 'ol' you can think of, makes sure that the pain is kept under control. Yes it still hurts like hell when I swallow, and swallowing is something I have to keep doing so that I don't forget how, but in general I am not in pain.

On that Thursday when I had to cancel my appointment at the hospital my neck was so sore that it made other people wince in pain for me. I was applying cream every couple of hours, and gel to the areas where the skin was breaking down. But on the following Monday morning I got up to find that a miracle had taken place overnight. The purpleness of my skin had toned down to pink, and the areas that had been cracked and bleeding had healed up overnight. All that was left was a dryness, not unlike when we get too much sun and our skin peels.

And from there on in, things are improving every day.

I still cannot swallow, I can't eat or drink even though I force myself to take a few sips of water every so often. It still hurts like hell to swallow, but I do it anyway because I know I have to. Yesterday I had six spoonfuls of chicken soup. It hurt, but I could taste it!

I was warned at the start of the treatment that I would lose all sense of taste, that my taste buds would be destroyed and that it could be up to a year before I get them back. But this doesn't seem to be the case. I am putting a small amount of orange cordial into my water, and I can taste this too. So perhaps I have been lucky; I won't know for certain until I am able to eat again.

I was also warned that I would be left with a permanent dry mouth at the end of the treatment. I don't know if this will be the case eventually, but for now it is not permanently dry, just some of the time.

If I were to be asked what the worst aspect of the treatment has been I would have to say it is the mucus that appears to be produced somewhere near the back of my throat. Strings of thick fluid, resembling spaghetti, that can only be cleared by spitting or by wiping away with strong tissue. I have found kitchen roll to be best for this job, and I make sure there is always plenty of this handy. Now, just over three weeks since the end of the treatment, even this is beginning to subside.

There are other things that are concerning me, some more than others.

When the last operation was performed Mr Small had to cut through a nerve to get to one of the glands that needed removing. This means that my tongue is now a rather odd shape and I have a bit of difficulty pronouncing my 's' sounds. I keep saying: sixty six sausages sizzling in the pan, but to my ears it doesn't sound right. Then again, this could have something to do with the mucus and my tongue could still be a little swollen from the treatment; time will tell.

The skin on my neck is ultra-sensitive. Where the operation was carried out, the surface flesh feels as though the nerves are exposed. It makes washing very difficult, and it makes my eyes pop out on stalks when my mother approaches me with her hands out.

Mum has a unique way of greeting those she loves; she puts out her hands and grabs either side of the neck, just under the ears, in a cupping the head gesture that is reserved for those who matter. As her memory is dreadful (nothing to do with her age, she just has a really bad memory), I have to keep jumping back and saying 'not the neck, don't touch the neck'.

2nd July 2009

Mum had an encounter with Mr Mian yesterday. Luckily Tom had also gone with her to what we had assumed would be a routine hospital visit, otherwise she would be very upset indeed now.

Bearing in mind that Mum in 82 years old, and a tad deaf, it's not difficult to work out that she might be in need of a little tenderness. Care and consideration has always been afforded to her at Barrow hospital prior to yesterday, and I am glad I can say that, other than Mr Mian, the medical staff at the hospital have always been kind to her, and have given her all the time and attention she has needed.

A few months ago a spot on Mum's forehead was bothering her a little, stinging when it was touched, and so she went to the doctor with it and was given an appointment to see a specialist at Barrow hospital. Tom went with her to this, and all subsequent appointments so we know that it's not just Mum getting confused. Mum was told that it was probably a form of skin cancer, and that it could be removed and that it was not something for her to worry about.

You have to remember that for people of my mother's age cancer is a dirty word; it is why I kept the extent of my condition from my parents for as long as possible. But the doctor she saw that day made sure that Mum understood that the condition she had was not life threatening.

A few weeks later she went in to hospital for a couple of hours, and the lump, and a couple of others she hadn't realised she had, was removed. The removal left her with big, black circles on her forehead and cheek, but she was assured, quite rightly, that these would disappear. Yesterday's visit was, as far as we were aware, just a check-up to make sure everything was ok.

Tom recognised Mr Mian from my description of him. Strong Indian accent, ostentatious gold watch, bruisk manner… it wasn't difficult for him to work out that this was the same man I had seen, the same man who had reduced me to tears.

'Ah, this is the lady with cancer,' was his opening greeting as my mother went into the room. They were words that sent a shiver of panic through Mum that showed in her eyes as she turned to look at Tom.

'Which side was the biopsy done?' He asked Mum, who pointed to where the spots had been removed. Had he bothered to take the time to read her notes he would have been already aware of where the procedure was carried out.

Tom told Mr Mian that the lumps had been removed, that it had not been biopsies. Again, something he could have determined for himself if he had taken the time to look.

Mr Mian was rough with my ageing mother, and the only time he smiled was when he asked her if she had any holidays planned over the next month and she told him, rather sadly in my opinion, that her days for holidays were over.

Now why was this a reason for Mr Mian to smile?

Unfortunately my Mum has to go back to see Mr Mian again because some cancerous cells were left when the last operations were done, so these have to be removed. And perhaps he is the best in his field in this area of the country, but I wish it were someone else doing the op on my Mum. She doesn't deserve his particular brand of bedside ill manner.

As for myself today; I have now got a rash on my face. It's not noticable, just a roughness across both cheeks, but again it's something new to contend with, and I shall. I had a good night's sleep, sleeping right through without needing a top up of drugs through the night to keep me in bed with morpheus.

Friday 3rd July 2009

Constipation is a harsh side effect of taking morphine. Anyone who thinks that they can take opiates and not suffer the dreadful curse of compacted faeces probably also buys regular lottery tickets.

I was provided with Movicol, a white powder that is mixed with water. Movicol is a stool softener, not a laxative, but getting the dosage right is nigh on impossible. But again, this is a small price to pay for being alive. At the moment I am using one sachet of Movicol per day, but it's not really enough, as my piles are witness to. But I know that two sachets is too much and leaves me with a fear of being any further than 50 yards away from a loo at any time. Perhaps I should try one and a half sachets… makes sense.

I seem to have woken on a downer this morning. It gets like this for me. Some days I feel as though I could take on anything; I feel positive and just know that I can get to the end of this and beat it into the ground. But not today; today I feel tired, not just physically but mentally too. My piles are sore, I am so thirsty and would love to be able to gulp back a long, cold drink, but my throat is mega sore, I am way too hot and I can't stop sneezing. The last thing I need right now is a cold, or worse still swine flu.

Swine flu is ravaging the country, and while the only people to die from it are people who are already incapacitated in some way, its still a worry. I wish people would stay away from the house until I know for sure I am fit enough to fight the flu; at the moment I don't feel fit enough to fight a fly.

I am tired of feeding via a tube. I tried soup again yesterday and managed to get ten spoonfuls inside me before the pain in my throat became too much to bear. Just what sort of damage does the radiotherapy do when four weeks after the end of the treatment, two weeks after the time when I am supposed to be healing, I am still in agony evey time I try to swallow?

I suppose I should be grateful that the pain is only there when I swallow; how unbearable would it be if that pain were there all of the time? I should also be grateful that I haven't suffered some of the side effects I was warned may happen, like a mouth full of blisters and sores. I put that down to the oral hygiene I implemented throughout my treatment. I used copious amounts of mouthwash, steralizing tablets for my falsies and made sure that my mouth was as clean as could be. And I am grateful not to be suffering these added extras, but that's not helping my mood today.

Could today's dark mood have anything to do with my visit to Mum and Dad yesterday? They are both in their eighties now, but while Mum (in spite of having to attend hospital for the skin cancer thing) is fit as a fiddle and bouncing, Dad is a physical wreck of his own making.

A few years ago Dad was found to have prostate cancer, and it seems that once told this he gave up and has done nothing but watch TV ever since, laid on the sofa, propped up by a cushion, in the same position day in, day out. He has laid there for so long that his body has now become stooped, his back permanently arced in the position he has taken up on the sofa. No amount of coaxing, cajoling or coercion can get him out of the house, and the only time he goes out is once a week to put on the lottery tickets and to purchase ridiculous amounts of scratch cards, still hoping for that big win he has hankered after all of his adult life.

Over a year ago he developed what is obviously a carcinoma on the outside of his ear. It sticks out at the top, like a little rubber duck aerial. Getting him to go to the doctor with it took months, and even when he did so and an appointment was arranged for him to see a specialist, he refused to go to hospital to have it removed because he is convinced that hospitals see off old folks with a pill. I'm not sure what this pill is supposed to be, nor where he has gathered his evidence from, but he would rather have a large, black growth on his ear than go to hospital to have it removed. He has been so stubborn about it that the specialist has arranged for the necessary equipment to be brought to this town, so that the procedure can be carried out here.

Dad also has a bad cough and at the same time as the specialist saw him about the lump on his ear an appointment was arranged for him to have a chest x-ray. But Dad refused to have this done, stating that if there was anything wrong then he didn't want to know. Curiously, he makes the journey to see the specialist looking after his prostate cancer without any complaints; he is going there today and doesn't mind at all. But when it comes to any other ailments, he simply buries his head in concrete and leaves it there.

He is sickeningly thin, weighing under 8 stone now, but he hardly eats at all, and when he does it is things like chocolate biscuits. There's no point in trying to force food on him, because he simply slides it off his plate when he thinks nobody is looking, wraps it in tissue and puts it into his pocket. Why he does this, why he doesn't want to eat… I wish I could fathom it. There was a time when he had a huge appetite, but now he hardly eats a thing. And yet he goes on about living to 100 as much as he ever has. Even when he was young, fit and healthy, he declared he intended to live to 100 so that he could get his telegram from the queen. He is nearly 86 now, 14 years to go, and unless a miracle happens, I doubt very much that we will be applying for that congratulatory message.

It's a huge worry, and yes I think it is possibly the cause of my black mood today. I know I have been lucky in that my parents have lived longer than any of their siblings and peers, and I know everyone has to go sometime. But the idea of my Mum being left on her own without the man that is her world… well, that thought just churns my stomach and I have no idea how I shall deal with it when the time comes. I hope I am wrong, I hope my Dad lives to 100 like he intends to; but I doubt it.

Saturday 4th July 2009

I think about death a lot more these days than I did prior to becoming ill. I say 'becoming ill' but to be honest I felt fine until the start of the treatment. All I had was some lumps on my neck, but because I didn't feel at all unwell I had presumed them to be cysts or something.

I am aware of my own mortality in a way I would rather not be. When I was younger mortality was just a word associated with how long people live, demographically speaking. But these days mortality is a word I associate with myself.

I can't say that I am any more scared of dying that I ever was. I'm not really scared of dying at all, after all it is something that comes to us all eventually. I *am* fearful of *how* I will die. This fear is at the root of other fears such as fear of flying and fear of being in vehicles on motorways. No, I am not more scared of dying, but I am more aware of death and all it means.

There was a time when I thought it really sad when someone died and nobody knew who they were. Like when old folks die alone and no relatives can be found and so only the funeral directors turn up to the service. I used to think how dreadfully sad it was that there was nobody there to mourn their passing, but now I think differently.

By far my biggest fear of death is leaving others to grieve. The idea of leaving this world before my mother fills me with dread. I cannot bear the notion of her being so heartbroken, as I know she would be, at the death of her only child.

Leaving my own children is another horror. I know that eventually the natural way of things is that parents die before their children, but they are not ready for me to go yet, and I don't want them to cry over me before they should. Heck, I don't want them to cry over me at all! Nor do I want my grandchildren upset at my passing, even though that will probably be the case one day; I just don't want it to be for a good number of years yet.

Man has been on this planet for millions of years (I think it's millions, but as I am no anthropologist please forgive me if I am wrong.) and yet we have never managed to get our heads around the fact that we all die eventually. Still funerals are full of people weeping and wailing, people who cannot believe that their loved ones are dead.

Whenever we are told that someone has died we look at the bearer of the news with astonishment and say 'No, really?' as though death is an ad-hoc event that only happens to the very unlucky. It's not a lottery; we all die, and it really is time that we started to get used to the idea.

The search for eternal life has been going on ever since the concept entered someone's head, and ever since then the marketing moguls have brainwashed generations of people, mostly women, into believing that looking younger is half the battle. Well it isn't!

Cosmetic surgery does not make people look younger, it simply makes them look as though they have had cosmetic surgery. Botox does not make people look younger, it simply makes them look as though they have had botox injections. And don't get me started on fake boobs.

Trying to make yourself look younger will not delay the ageing process, and nor will it postpone death when it comes calling. I'm not suggesting that everyone should give up on trying to look nice, I'm just saying that preoccupation with looking younger will do nothing to hinder the onset of age. We all get older, just as we all die, and we can do that with dignity, or we can go down the cosmetic surgery route and end up looking like Sly Stalone's mother. Enough said.

Most people have a 'things to do before I die' list, even if that list is only held on a mental clipboard. The BBC held a survey to find out what most people have on this list, and top of all came 'swim with dolphins'.

Why?

Out of all the things I would like to do before I die, swimming with fish is not one of them. Ok, so dolphins are technically mammals, that's not the point. They are fish shaped, they live in the sea and they swim a lot. What is the attraction?

Running with a cheetah… now there would be an ambition. Not that it's one of mine. But if you really have to top your list with emulating the characteristics of a wild creature, why not make it something interesting?

Playing a round of golf at Augusta, Georgia, USA is another one that made it into the BBC top 50 things to do before I die list. I reckon that's another one that will never make it to my list. I'm with whoever said that golf is a good walk ruined.

However, there are things on the list that I have on my own mental list before I ever Googled the subject. Things like; gallop a horse along a beach, which is a rather odd thing for me to have on my list as I am terrified of horses. Oh and a best-selling novel or two would be nice.

I once had a friend who worked with horses and one day I sat next to her on the bus coming home from town and remarked on the huge bruise on the top of her arm. I didn't remark on the smell that eminated from her, that was something that came with the job of working with horses and it would have been impolite to say 'God, what's that awful stench?'

'Bonny bit me this afternoon,' she explained with a chuckle.

I looked at the bruise again. Now, Barbara was a horsey kind of girl, built for pushing horses back into place when they got out of line, and as such she had developed rather large arms over the years. So this was no small bruise, this was no little nip, this bruise covered the spectrum and every inch of the top of Barbara's arm.

'Horses bite?' I recall being quite shocked to learn this as Barbara laughed and said 'Of course they do.' as she initiated my fear of horses. Hence, I have never got close to one ever since then; and that incident was some 40 years ago.

But still, overcoming fears is what challenges are all about, and I would love to try horse riding before I die. So when I mentioned it to my granddaughter and she pointed out that she too is scared of horses, so this is why I suggested that we overcome our fear together sometime. She agreed readily, so perhaps it may happen one day.

The reason behind my wish to fly to New York is to ride in a yellow cab. But again, I'm not sure that will ever happen as to get there I would have to fly to America, and that's one heck of a long flight. I can just about cope with a flight to Dublin, which takes around 30 minutes, so I'm not really sure that I could fly all the way to the states. Although, it's not really a problem I am every likely to face as I can't afford to go.

Singing backing vocals for David Bowie; another of my dreams that is unlikely to come to fruition. David is considerably older than me, and therefore is likely to die before me. Not only that, there are lots of other obstacles standing in the way of my carrying out this particular 'thing to do before I die'. At the moment I can't sing; a matter that is deeply concerning to me. I mentioned this to my daughter in law and she said I should think myself lucky, that she has *never* been able to sing. When I try to sing now all that comes out is a strange vibrato noise, which I am sure Mr Bowie would not find remotely attractive as a backing sound to Golden Years. My singing voice makes me sound like a Dalek, and is not exactly tuneful.

In case you haven't noticed, I'm feeling a lot better today. I slept through the night again without having to get up to take pain killers, and while I still can't eat or drink because it's far too painful to swallow, I feel a lot more positive than I did going to bed last night.

Sunday 5th July 2009

And today I feel like shit!

This treatment (torture) really is a roller coaster of feelings, emotions and temperament. I got through most of yesterday feeling fine, apart from being pissed off at not being able to drink something long and cool on such a hot day. Today I woke up fit to strangle; specifically, my next door neighbour who seems to think that she lives in a detached house in the middle of nowhere and that there couldn't possibly be anyone trying to sleep on the other side of the wall at 8.00 am on a Sunday morning.

She has lived there for several years now, and yet she has still not got the hang of closing her back door without slamming it several times first. Slamming it obviously does not work, so why doesn't she go straight for whatever it is that she does when she closes it on the third, fourth or fifth attempt?

Yes, I think my neighbour waking me so early has something to do with my mood today; let's hope it lightens as the day goes on. I also feel a little sick this morning, and that's going to have to clear up for my mood to lighten in any way.

The boredom is driving me a little crazy. Because my mind has been taken over by Morpheus and his minions I find it difficult to concentrate on anything for very long. Once the drugs kick in all I really want to do is sleep; which is why I write this first thing in the morning, before my eyes start to shut of their own accord.

I have been trying to contact Eddie and Val by email, but I think I must have their address wrong because I'm not getting any reply. I really would like to know how Eddie is getting on; perhaps I will bump into them sometime at the hospital.

Monday 6th July 2009

When all this started, early in this year, I had it in my head that it would take about 3 weeks for the surgery and recovery, followed by 3 weeks for the radiotherapy, and then I would be back at work. And before that I would have said I was a pesamist rather than an optimist. By my calculations I should have been back at work by the end of April. But as you can see it is now July, and there is no sign of my being able to go back to work yet.

I tried to eat some cold custard yesterday. I could taste it, in a vague sort of way, which is good, and means that my taste buds are working a bit, but after swallowing about 3 spoonfulls my throat felt like it was being scraped by barbed wire and I had to stop. It is so depressing when I try to eat and cannot because the pain is too intense. But I suppose that cancer and depression go hand in hand, at some level. Surely nobody can be told they have cancer and still stay completely optimistic and cheerful.

I am scared. I cannot deny that. Every moment of every day, no matter what I am doing, no matter what conversations I may be having with anyone, the fear of the cancer is still at the back of my mind. Perhaps because my cancer is hidden it makes it all the worse. If the scans had shown a tumor that the radiotherapy could have been aimed at, if subsequent scans showed that the tumor had been killed off; perhaps then I could relax in the knowledge that my cancer had been dealt with. But that will never be the case for me.

The radiotherapy I went through was so intense and so aggressive because the doctors wanted to make sure that they hit their hidden target. They know it's there somewhere, so if they hit everything they have to get it. That's the theory anyway. But the only way I will know that they have definitely got their 'man' will be if no more lumps come up. That's the fear I am going to have to live with; the fear of finding more lumps.

I know that I can never have radiotherapy in that area again. Dr Siva has made that very clear. It is not possible because to do so would put more strain on my spinal cord than it could take, and I could end up completely paralysed if more radiotherapy were carried out. So if I ever do develop more lumps... what then? I am sure you can understand why I am left with a deep set paranoia.

Oh dear; I started writing this with the intention of keeping the content as light hearted as possible. However, as I have worked on it I have found that it is not possible to keep a book such as this light hearted all of the time. Yes there are aspects of my journey through cancer that have been amusing, and I hope that I have raised a smile, or even a chuckle, or two along the way. But I cannot apologise for there being a dark side to my story. Cancer is a dark subject; and no matter what advances are made in diagnostics and cures I suspect it will be many a year before a cure for every cancer is found and the fear is a thing of the past.

I truly believe that one day people will read works such as this and feel nothing but pity for people like me, people who have to go through torturous treatments such as radiotherapy and chemotherapy. In the future people will be cured of cancer as easily as people are cured of other illnesses today, illnesses that once killed people. There was a time when diarrhea would kill people, but today we just pop to the chemist and get something for it without even having to see a docotor, and I really believe that one day cancer will be treated in a similar simple fashion.

Wednesday 8th July 2009

I had another check-up at Preston yesterday. Mr Small wasn't there, so Dr Siva was the one responsible for putting the camera up my nose to see how things are going on down there. I could have looked at the screen to see for myself, but I chose not to, some things in life you just don't want to see, and my ulcerous throat is one of them.

Dr Siva was happy with what he saw, and that's the main thing. While my throat is still covered in ulcers, it is starting to heal, and he is happy with my progress. I wish I was.

For me the progress is torturously slow. Again last night I tried to eat something, this time soup from a corned beef hash. One mouthful was all I managed; it stung like crazy and there was no point in putting myself through agony to try to get more down. There was probably pepper in it, and I can't imagine my throat coping too well with pepper at this stage.

But what stage? What stage am I at now?

I am over the fear of the treatment, the fear that prompted me to write this in the first place. I had to write about my fear because I couldn't say to people 'Oh my god, I am so scared my head is spinning off my shoulders.' But as time went on, and as I climbed carefully over every hurdle that was placed in front of me, this fear gave way to determination; determination that I was going to get through the treatment and see it through to the very end. And I did that; there was not a single day during the treatment that I did not turn up for radiotherapy and chemotherapy. That's not to say that I didn't want to bury my head under the duvet and tell the world to go away, that

I couldn't cope any more; of course I felt like that, I'm no hero, but I did it all regardless. Then the last day of treatment came, and I began to dread the next couple of weeks. I knew that the radiotherapy went on working inside the body even after the treatment was finished, and by that stage I felt so ill that I really didn't think I would be able to cope with what was to come.

But I had to; there was no turning back; there was no saying 'No thank you, I don't want to do that today.' because it was already done. I remember having similar feelings while in labour with my first child; this was something that I could not run away from, could not change my mind about; whatever my feelings, it was all going to happen, regardless.

I was right to dread those two weeks; there's no point in dressing it up as anything other than the trial it was. My neck was so sore that it split and cracked, I threw up without any notice and I felt so ill that all I wanted to do was sleep. But eventually even that started to get better. The getting better part happens so slowly that it is not possible to define a particular time when particular healing occurs.

Right now I know that I still have a long way to go. My throat is still so sore that I cannot eat or drink, so I am still feeding through the tube in my belly. That's the next fear I have to face, having the tube removed. I asked a nurse what it was like to have it removed and she told me it was like being kicked; but she didn't say by what; an elephant, a horse, a hamster... whatever, I am still dreading it, although I have to say, I would much prefer it to be the latter. But knowing my luck it will be like being kicked by an elephant. Whatever, I will report it here at a later date.

I don't know if there's much point in trying to write this every day now. Perhaps I should leave it until something significant happens, like having the tube removed.

We'll see, as my Dad always said when I was a little girl and he couldn't answer whatever question I had put to him.

Thursday 9th July 2009

And just a day later here I am.

Chocolate mousse brought me back; the chocolate mousse made with hot chilies. Well, to be honest, the list of ingredients says nothing about chilies. I had decided that I could eat chocolate mousse; why not? If I could cope with half a cup of chicken soup, as I had done yesterday afternoon, then there was no reason why I couldn't cope with chocolate mousse, after all, it's only flavoured air… or so I thought.

Yes, I could taste it. As I put half a teaspoonful of mousse on my tongue the chocolate flavour enveloped my senses and sent me to chocolate heaven, for a second, and then I swallowed.

Oh boy, that hurt like I cannot tell you. I don't know what was in that mousse but once it hit the back of my throat I was in agony. Since when did they start to make chocolate mousse with drain cleaner?

Half a bloody teaspoonful, that's all I ate of the mousse that was going to be mannah to me. It was going to be God sent food and I was going to live on it until I could cope with other foods. But the God of Oh Really… he said no!

Friday 10th July 2009

Another strange side effect of taking so much morphine are the dreams that come every night.

I have been abducted by aliens so many times that I have to wonder if this is a hidden fear of mine that only comes out I dreams. I recall a conversation with Dan at work; Dan said he relished the idea of aliens from another world coming to Earth, whereas I had to admit that the thought quite terrified me. So perhaps it *is* a hidden fear that only comes to the surface of my consciousness while I am asleep.

Friday 17th July 2009

Over a month since the completion of the treatment, and I really thought I would be eating by now, but progress is slow, so slow that I hardly notice it happening, yet it is. A few weeks ago I struggled to get sips of water down my throat, now I am struggling to get certain soft foods down.

I haven't tried the drain cleaner/chocolate mousse again, but chicken soup goes down fairly well. When I say fairly well, I don't mean that I can swallow it without any problems, but that I can swallow it with less problems than other foods. I thought I would be able to cope with Minestrone soup if I put it through a strainer, but no, it was agony due to the amount of pepper it contained. Then I decided to try mash (the instant variety) with corned beef mashed into it. This didn't hurt like the minestrone soup, but it stuck to the inside of my mouth like strong wallpaper paste. I have the same problem with chocolate. The dry mouth will not allow the consumption of a tiny piece of chocolate. It sticks to the inside of my mouth and has to be washed away with water. It's so damned uncomfortable that I doubt I will ever eat chocolate again.

Last night I tried cornflakes with warm milk. I let the cornflakes get really soggy before trying to eat them, and while it was not a pain free experience, I did manage to get them down by following spoonfuls of cornflakes with sips of cold water. I am just about to try Ready Brek, so I will be back in a short while with a report on how that went. I was waiting for the meds to kick in before trying.

And done; I got it all down eventually. It took about a quarter of an hour to consume a couple of serving spoons full of Ready Brek, and it hurt a bit, but it's in my tummy now, so if necessary I could survive on chicken soup and Ready Brek.

A catastrophe occurred the other night, my tube broke. The end of the tube just fell off in my hand and I went into a small panic, actually, it was a rather large panic. At the time I was only getting chicken soup into me, and only small amounts at that, and I couldn't see how I could possibly survive on nothing but chicken soup if I couldn't get the Ensures down the tube. One thing I knew for sure, there was no way I was having another tube fitted unless they knocked me out first, so if I couldn't fix the tube it was chicken soup or nothing.

Out came the gaffer tape (duck tape) and I repaired the tube with several small strips that have held for over 48 hours now. I may have to repeat the repair before the tube is eventually removed, but I would rather repair it before every feed rather than have a new one fitted.

Sunday 19th July 2009

Coffee makes me cough. How very strange.

I can drink water without any problems now, I can also drink tea, but coffee makes me cough as soon as it hits the back of my throat.

Yesterday I ate half a can of macaroni cheese. Yes I know, I could have made my own, but my train of thought was that if I went to all the trouble of making cheese sauce and then I couldn't eat it… well, how annoying would that be? So it made more sense to buy it in a can. It hurt to get it down, but I coped. Later I tried peaches and cream. Curiously, although I find I can taste most foods that I try, peaches and cream was almost completely tasteless to me. But again, with perseverance, I managed to get three slices of peach into my stomach.

Progress is very, very slow, but I have to keep trying, even when I really don't want to.

Tuesday 21ˢᵗ July 2009

I had to go to see Doctor Walker yesterday as I woke up really hoarse and my throat was rather sore. I didn't really want to go around to the surgery because I had heard that someone had been there on Friday and had been diagnosed with swine flu. In my over active imagination swine flu germs would be clinging to every surface, and would pounce on me the moment I went through the door of the surgery.

Swine flu is ravaging the country at the moment, and the population is in a state of panic despite the fact that the only deaths that have occurred have been in people who have had underlying medical problems, mainly heart defects. While it has now been over six weeks since the completion of my treatment, I'm not sure if my immune system has built itself back up to a level that could cope with flu, swine or otherwise. I certainly don't want to have to cope with the effects of flu, not hot on the heels of the effects of radiotherapy.

It turned out that I have a touch of thrush at the back of my throat, and Dr Walker gave me medication for that. Also, he thinks I may have been overdoing it on the eating front. Eating Ready Brek, macaroni cheese and peaches and cream may have been a bit too much for one day. He explained that inside my throat is hard scar tissue, like a scab, and that when this is damaged it cracks and can be very painful. So when I have my Ready Brek today I will make sure it is good and sloppy. I was also wondering if baby rice might be a good idea; after all, this is designed to give babies a healthy, nutritional meal.

This morning I had a look at the online newspaper report on the man who has swine flu in this town. He went to the doctor's on Friday and it was confirmed that he had this particular nasty strain of the virus.

Then I got to wondering how? How exactly did the doctor he saw deduce that the man had swine flu? If he/she were just basing his diagnosis on a list of symptoms then the man could have had any number of things wrong with him. Without blood tests it is not possible to know for sure that swine flu was the cause of the man's illness.

I have decided to panic no longer.

I am still worrying about other things though.

I know that my boss has told me not to worry about getting back to work until I am recovered, but still I am concerned that I will have forgotten all of my training by the time I get back. Not only that, but money is going to be very tight very soon if I don't get back to work. So what is stopping me from going back?

I can't speak properly yet. My throat is preventing me from talking without sounding hoarse when I do it for too long. So talking on the phone all day would be out of the question right now.

The PEG feeding tube is still attached to my stomach, through which most of my sustenance and medication goes. To be able to do lunch at work I would need a room where I could lock myself away to pour an Ensure down my tube.

The medication makes me sleepy. Every afternoon I go for a nap for two to three hours. While I would be happy to come off the medication tomorrow I know this is not possible because the pain in my throat would be very severe without it, and morphine is not a drug that anyone can simply stop taking. I will have to be weaned off it, gradually reducing the amount I take, because to just stop would be to induce the DTs, or so I am told.

But it is now late July, and I had hoped to be back at work by September. At the moment I'm not sure if this is going to happen. I had not expected the healing process to take so long. I had based my estimation on how long it takes for a sore to heal on the skin, and it is now apparent that the sores down my throat will take much longer than a flesh wound to heal.

At least I am not smoking, because I can't imagine how much longer the healing process would take if I were to be torturing my throat with hot smoke. I have got to a stage now where I hate smoking with a passion. I have gone from being one of the heaviest smokers I knew, to despising everything about tobacco; I hate the smell, the cost, the damage it does to people's health… everything about smoking is abhorrent to me now, and I hope it stays that way. Smoking is not really a choice once you start, cigarettes have a hold on people like no other drug. Yes, the first time a person smokes it is by choice, but later on, when the tobacco has taken hold, it is like trying to get out of the grip of a vice. I know of people who have come off heroin but still they can't give up smoking.

Big Brother is on TV at the moment; some love it, some hate it. I am in the former category. I love to watch the personalities of the 'contestants' develop over the weeks. For anyone with an interest in people, and the psychology that makes people tick, Big Brother is like a living thesis.

While a few of the contestants this year smoke, two in particular, Karly and Lisa, have serious addictions. Their need for tobacco is so bad that when they failed the shopping task and were given a basic budget of £1 per head per day to live on, both Karly and Lisa purchased tobacco instead of food, declaring that they would rather live off lentils and chick peas than give up their cigarettes. Perhaps when they see how pathetic they appeared they may decide to take control of their addictions, because they came across as junkies, desperate for their fix. To see Karly go through the ashtray, desperately scavenging for old dog ends, which she then smoked… it was disgusting. It was so vile that this footage should be shown in schools, to children who have not yet started to smoke as it would put anyone off.

Thursday 23rd July 2009

Coffee still makes me cough, I don't know why. But this morning I got up with a determination to have a cup of coffee in an attempt to kick start normality in my life. And in a little while I am going to have Ready Brek for breakfast and I am going to take my medication orally. I took my medication orally last night and although the oramorph stung a little as it went down my throat, it was bearable. I am so tired of this tube in my stomach and I so want rid of it, but I know that the only way this is going to happen is if I am taking enough food through my mouth to be able to sustain me. Because my throat has been a little hoarse I haven't been eating food, but yesterday I took my Ensures orally, and I intend to do the same today. It is my intention that as soon as I have gone a whole week without using the tube I will ask to have it removed.

I know it's going to hurt, but whatever it feels like, it will only be for a brief moment, and then my stomach will be my own again. If there ever came a time when I had a need to have a feeding tube inserted again for any reason, I think I would prefer to have the one that goes down the nose. It may look a little unsightly, but the trauma of having this one fitted is something I don't think I could ever go through again.

Friday 24th July 2009

I managed to get through the whole day without using my tube yesterday. The only food I ate was Ready Brek. At teatime I decided to try some ravioli, the tinned variety. As with the macaroni cheese I had no intention of going to the trouble of making it from scratch, in case I couldn't eat it. Who am I kidding? I have never made ravioli from scratch in my life. The closest I have got to cooking fresh pasta is to buy those little pasta parcels at the supermarket. I wouldn't have a clue how to make fresh pasta.

Disappointingly, the ravioli tasted awful, and so I had a strawberry flavoured Ensure instead. And it was then that I started to feel really down as I began to wonder just what my diet is going to consist of in the future.

Yes I am alive, and that was the whole point of the treatment. But I have to wonder just how that life is now changed. I asked Jane how David copes with eating and she told me that the only thing he can't really eat is cream crackers, so that gave me hope. But, of course, everyone is different, and I have no idea how I am going to cope with eating in the future.

Already I know that eating chocolate is out of the question. This has nothing to do with my throat being sore, but because of the dry mouth. Chocolate will not move along and sticks to the inside of my mouth. Potatoes do the same thing. And so I started to feel rather depressed last night, realising I will probably have to go through life without ever eating another Cadbury's Cream Egg.

How sad is that? I don't mean how sad is it that I won't be eating my favourite sticky confectionary again; I mean how sad is it that I seem to be measuring quality of life with chocolate and potatoes? There are people in this world who have lived their life with no knowledge whatsoever of a cream egg; and until a few hundred years ago potatoes had never been heard of in this country.

I really need to get my head around the idea that my personal menu has now changed. I have to get used to the idea that I will not be able to eat certain foods, things such as biscuits, and get on with working out exactly what I will be able to eat.

At the moment my taste buds are not cooperating fully with my dietary decisions; some foods I can taste, some I can't, some taste strange. But eventually my taste buds will be back to normal and I will be able to enjoy Heinz's ravioli again. Although I can eat Ready Brek without any difficulties, no matter how much sugar I put in it, it still doesn't taste sweet. I couldn't taste the peaches and cream either, so I wonder if it is a problem with sweet tastes that I am having at the moment.

There should be a list of foods that can be eaten easily with a dry mouth; perhaps I should put one together for people who have to go through the same treatment that I have just been through. It seems to be a fairly common treatment, and yet there is no list of foods that are easy to consume with a dry mouth, which is a certain consequence of head and neck radiotherapy.

Today I am as determined as ever to get through without using my tube. I have yet to eat anything, but that's because I'm not hungry, not because of any fear of pain. It seems as though the pain has subsided greatly and once again I have taken my medication orally.

It is seven weeks today since I received my last session of radiotherapy, and only today that I can report I am just about free of pain in my throat and can swallow without wincing. I wince when I swallow the oramorph, but that's just because it is like a shot of strong spirits, not because it hurts to swallow it. I follow it with the dissolvable slow release morphine and that washes away any bad taste that may be left. I find it really peculiar that so many strong medicines, like morphine and voltarol, are fruit flavoured and taste quite nice. If any child were to get their hands on such medication they could easily swallow it. Not that this would happen in my house, but it's not difficult to see how this could happen.

Saturday 25th July 2009

Day two without using the tube for feeding, and now the weight loss is starting, but this is unavoidable really.

I was told at the start of my treatment that I was likely to lose weight, and anywhere I looked online, people who had gone through this treatment stated that they had lost a lot of weight. For me, this was the one consolation, having put on nearly three stone over the past few years since I had my hysterectomy. But it didn't happen, not in any significant way. When I first started to use the tube I lost about half a stone, but because I began feeding with the Ensures as soon as I realised I was struggling to eat normally, I didn't lose a lot of weight. But now that I have started to try to eat regular food I am losing weight at a rather rapid rate. This week alone I have lost five pounds.

Yesterday I tried eating some scrambled egg, but while I would have eaten at least two eggs in no time at all prior to the radiotherapy, I only managed to eat about half of one egg yesterday, and that took around a quarter of an hour to get down. Today I am going to try an omelette, just with one egg, perhaps that will be a bit tastier.

I didn't just eat part of one egg yesterday, that would be silly. I also had a bowl of Ready Brek and a couple of Ensures, but I wasn't very hungry. It really is getting me down that I can't eat what I want when I want. That's the spoiled westerner in me. I know I should be grateful that I can eat at all, and I know there are many people in this world who would happily live on scrambled egg and Ready Brek for the rest of their lives and still feel grateful, just to be alive.

Someone on TV last night said how nice it is to go out and do the shopping and to have a fridge full off food to choose from. When this was said I imagined my fridge full of milk and eggs. I have no doubt that as time goes on I will discover more and more foods that I can eat, that I can fill the fridge with, but at the moment I am struggling. As usual, I want to run before I can walk. My throat is only starting to get better and I expect to be able to eat a three course meal with cheese and biscuits at the end.

Cheese, another of my favourite foods. I tried to eat the smallest sliver of cheese the other night, but it wouldn't go down and I ended up having to spit it out. Perhaps I will be able to eat cream cheese, but the cheese that I love, mature Cheddar, will be out of the question as my dry mouth will not cooperate with mastication.

Another idea I had last night was to try opal fruits, or starburst as they are now called. Everyone knows that just the thought of eating opal fruits is enough to get the saliva glands working overtime. I don't need mine to work overtime, I just need them to work enough to allow me to eat dry foods. But nothing happened other than the fact that the first sweet I tried got stuck in my mouth and when I finally retrieved it from my teeth I gave it to the dog. She doesn't mind if her food has been previously chewed. I really have to stop giving her things that I can't eat or she is going to turn into a coffee table dog.

Speaking of coffee. I don't think that it is the coffee itself that is making me cough, I think it is the milkyness. The Ensures do the same thing. I don't think it is anything to do with milk itself, but the milky texture. I'm going to try a cup of black coffee today, and if I can get that down without coughing I will try to get used to drinking coffee without milk.

I wish I didn't live in this grim little northern town where there is nothing to do. If I were in Dublin I could get ready and go into town, not necessarily to buy anything, just to soak up the atmosphere of the city, to wander around the shops, to listen to the buskers and to sit in St Stephen's green watching the world go by as I wonder what people do for a living, where they are going etc. But here there is only one street of shops, and the only park is a hill covered in grass with a kiddie's play area in the middle. There is an area at the end of my street that is laughingly called a 'nature reserve', but in reality this is the slag bank from the town's mining days that has overgrown with grass and weeds. The only signs of nature are the rabbits that can be heard running for cover into the bushes whenever anyone passes by.

I was awake early this morning. At the back of my house is another area where 'nature' is nurtured; in the form of allotments that have been there for many, many years. But I wouldn't mind if these allotments were used for growing food. There is one fool who has a pigeon loft out there, some 50 feet away from my house, and most mornings he is out there banging and scraping, but today, as on many mornings, he was calling in the pigeons with his incessant 'come on, come on, come on...' until I want to scream. These birds have flown home from god knows where, but this idiot believes that without his constant yelling they will never make it the twenty yards or so from the sky to their home. He calls them from where he sits, on an office chair that he has fixed to the roof of his shed. It is the most bizarre thing to see. Right in the middle of the allotments, an office chair nailed to a roof.

So, because of this idiot I have a long day to fill. If I didn't have this stupid tube attached to my stomach I would take a long bath. But because I keep forgetting to ask if I can have a bath with it still there, I have only dared to shower of late. I don't know what I imagine is going to happen if I have a bath; will my stomach fill with bath water?

The wound area where the tube is fitted has never healed properly. Many years ago I had my ears pierced, but eventually I had to concede that my body was never going to accept the foreign objects that I put in these holes. Every time I tried to wear earrings the holes would become infected, and it is much the same with the hole that the tube pokes through.

About a week after the tube was fitted it started to weep green gunge, and it has continued to do so ever since. I have to keep a dressing around it to soak up the seepage, and I doubt very much if the wound would heal if the tube were there until the end of my days.

It doesn't seem to bother the medical staff; I have shown it to several doctors and nurses but they don't appear to be concerned about it. I have been told that if it starts to weep puss it will be a different matter (no pun intended). Apparently puss *is* a different matter to what is seeping from the wound now. Puss smells, but whatever is coming from it at the moment doesn't. I have had a couple of courses of anti biotics to try to clear it up, but nothing has worked, so I just continue to try to keep the area clean.

My body's reaction to the tube is probably not the norm. I know that Eddie, who had the same tube fitted, didn't have any problems once it had been in a few weeks. I wonder how he and Val are getting on. I tried to email them at the address they gave me, but I have not received a reply, so I wonder if it were wrong. That said, I gave them my email address but haven't received anything from them that way either. Perhaps ours was just one of those hospital relationships that wasn't meant to go on any longer. Shame, because I really liked the pair of them and would like to know how Eddie is doing, especially if he is doing really well.

There are two people in my street that have had cancer diagnosed recently. One is an elderly man who has been told he has about three months left to live; the other has been informed that he has probably had his cancer for years without knowing about it, but is going for treatment so I am keeping my fingers crossed for him that he will be made well.

My mother also has to go into hospital next week for further treatment. She had those lumps taken from her head, but now it is feared that the surrounding areas still have some cells that need to be got rid of, so she is going in overnight to have this done. It's only a small operation, but she is in her eighties, and I would rather she didn't have to face this. Then again, I would prefer my mother to go on living her active life, so it is a necessary evil that the operation is carried out.

It is being done by Mr Mian. As you can imagine I'm not exactly thrilled that he is performing the operation, but apparently he is very good at what he does, even if he has no people skills, so I assume my mother to be in good hands, from a surgical point of view.

Dad doesn't think Mum needs to have the operation done at all. He can't understand why she has to go into hospital when she 'looks fine', as he pointed out to me last week. Unfortunately Dad has got it into his head that the only reason old people are taken into hospital is so that they can be given a little white pill (why white?… ask my Dad) and killed off. He's not specific about what is in this little white pill, but I assume it to be something to make the old person die quietly, some sort of very strong sleeping pill from which the elderly cannot wake. But I have faith that Mum will be fine.

I have sat here writing this for over an hour, and completely forgot to take my medication. That has to be a sign that I am really on the road to recovery. It's only a few weeks ago that I was getting up in the middle of the night to take painkillers, just so that I could sleep fitfully. Now I am sleeping right through, and am in so little pain that I forgot I needed to take anything for it. I really must be careful. I have been told that if I just stop taking the morphine that I could end up suffering withdrawal symptoms, which apparently are like flu symptoms, and with swine flu so prevalent at the moment, I really don't need that kind of panic.

Sunday 26th July 2009

Whether or not it is part of the illness, a reaction to the drugs or part of the treatment, and its subsequent effects, I don't know. But this morning I awoke feeling horribly depressed; a 'where is my life going' feeling that I am finding difficult to shake off. Looking back at what I wrote yesterday, I can see that this feeling was starting to build up then. I could do with someone to talk to about it, but who? Tom is happy at the moment, he just got himself a new motorbike and is so excited about it that I'm not about to bring him down from his happy cloud by telling him I feel really miserable.

I wish I was into motorbikes and that I wasn't shit scared of getting on the back of it, but I am. If I were not scared of it we could go off for days out on it at the weekends. It's not Tom's first bike, and there was a time when I wasn't such a wuss and we would go off to the lakes together, or visit little villages and have something to eat. When I was younger I didn't have the fears I have now; I was able to shrug off the 'I don't want to end up a mangled mess' feeling by telling myself that Tom was a good driver and that these things happened to other people. But then, I also felt the same about cancer; that was something that happened to others. Over the years I have come to realise that all things are possible. I feel as though I have just been handed back my life, and I don't want to take any chances with it.

There was a time when I would pop next door and talk my feelings out with a friend, but that was when I lived in Ireland. Although I have lived in this street for fifteen years, there is nobody I can drop in on for the craic. I know everyone to say hello to, and even to stop and have a chat with in the street. But nobody ever says: 'drop in for a coffee', nobody socialises, everyone lives their own lives behind closed doors. The friends I have had in this town have all left, bar one, and she lives about two miles away and works all hours of the day, and sometimes through the night. I have no social life whatsoever. The last time I had a night out was when I was in Dublin just before the start of the treatment; the time before that was last August when we celebrated my parents' diamond wedding anniversary.

Perhaps this is why I miss work so much. I work with a bunch of intelligent, quick witted people, and I really enjoy spending time with them. Sadly, work has become my social life, and being stuck at home... I miss it.

I know what you're thinking; get out and do something about it. But what? I don't want to sit in local pubs, playing dominoes and bingo with people who knit their own cardigans. There are no decent restaurants to go and have a nice meal in, even if I could eat. I'm hardly Women's Institute material and I don't fancy playing bowls. I'm way too old to go to nightclubs at the weekend; besides which, I have no longing to spend my time surrounded by drunken teenagers and people who have yet to realise that *they* are too old for nightclubs.

On Monday mornings people at work ask 'Nice weekend Lynn?' and I reply 'Quiet.' I give the same response to queries about how Christmas went and how holiday time was spent. Everything in my life is quiet now. Saturdays are spent getting my clothes ready for the week ahead and catching up on correspondence; Sundays are spent trying to entertain my elderly parents. I never go anywhere or do anything.

Yesterday, when Tom went to buy his bike I tried to fill up the day, but I just didn't know how. I walked up to the supermarket and bought a couple of tins of soup and some jelly; then I walked back home again, looking in the shop windows along the way; shops that sell sheets and curtains, electrical goods and household objects. I knew that if I were in Dublin I would have friends to call in on, or I could get the bus into town and wander around shops with exciting window displays; or I could just sit in St Stephen's Green and watch the world go by. But here there is nothing, and I spent the day alone, watching TV or napping until there was a knock on the door early evening and my daughter in law was standing there with my little grandson in her arms. Then life took on a different feel. We walked to the play park and I took delight from watching my grandson play; chuckling and giggling, toddling from one thing to another in his fascination.

I feel so isolated in this town; isolated and insular. If we lived in Barrow I would have lots of people I could socialise with; people from work who are always asking me along to their nights out. I could spend time with our kids and their children… there is so much I could do if only I was not stuck in this 'quiet' town.

And I hear you; do something about it… move to Barrow. And I almost growl in frustration. Yes I know… I would love to. But to do so would mean selling my house and buying another, and at the moment house prices have plummeted so much that I would find it very difficult to sell, and then I would have to find another one to buy, and at my age I am not sure I would be able to transfer my mortgage over. Besides which, I cannot leave my parents here on their own.

Dad can hardly walk, and has to get a taxi even to come to my house, and I am only a five minute walk away. And while Mum is still quite sprightly for her age, I could hardly move away and leave her on her own. No, for now I am stuck here in this apathetic little town where lack of ambition or imagination is indigenous. The sooner I get back to work the better. Were it not for the Internet for entertainment I think I would surely go mad.

Well, that was a little rant wasn't it? But this is a diary after all, of sorts, and if I can't put my feelings down here, where can I put them? I miss Ireland, I miss the wit and the craic, and I would go back tomorrow if I could bring my entire family with me. Everyone knows I miss Ireland, I don't make any secret of it, but today it is a burning feeling in the pit of my stomach. Today I could happily get on a plane and go to Dublin, just for the day.

Perhaps these strong feelings of depression have something to do with the drugs I am taking; after all, have you ever seen a happy junkie? They always look miserable; so perhaps it is the morphine; perhaps when I get off it completely I will cheer up.

As for how I am doing physically; yesterday I ate half a can of tomato soup and half a pot of strawberry jelly. Other than that I got a few of Ensures down my neck as well to top up the calories I need to keep me going. I also ate a chip (yes, just one chip) washed down with plenty of water, and a sliver of gammon. This morning I coughed up a small bit of the gammon that had been lodged at the back of my throat all night. So I guess I shouldn't be eating foods like that just yet. I just wanted the taste.

It is almost two months since the end of the treatment, and still I am not able to eat anything other than liquid foods such as soup, or slimy food like macaroni cheese. And even these simple foods take forever to get down. I long for the day when I can eat solids again, but I have not been told when that is likely to be.

The annual Flookborough Steam Gathering is taking place today. Flookborough is about thirty miles away from here and the gathering of steam engines is a highlight of the social calendar in these parts. My son and his wife are going, because her father builds steam engines (which may sound boring but the miniature engine he shows at such gatherings really is amazing) but I decided not to go for two reasons. Firstly, call me tight but a £10 entrance fee seems a bit steep to me. Secondly; there are burger and hot dog stalls all over the place, and the smell of the food would be tormenting.

But this morning, when I woke feeling so down I decided it might be a good idea to go after all. So what if I had to put up with the tormenting smells of cooking; I cope when people have barbeques locally. But I pulled back the curtains, and as though the weather has changed to match my mood, it is pouring down with rain. The beautiful blue sky from yesterday has been obliterated by grey clouds, and although the birds are still twittering outside my house (smiles at the thought of birds at computers) I don't think it's with happiness.

Perhaps the god of 'Oh Really' is as disgusted as I am at the £10 entrance fee the organisers have decided to charge this year. Perhaps when they rubbed their hands together with glee at the amount of money they were going to make he looked down and said: 'Oh Really!' Usually hundreds of people turn up for the gathering. It's not only steam engines but there are also lots of stalls and all manner of country type things going on, so it is generally very entertaining. But not this year; only the very brave and dedicated are likely to turn up today. Not many people are going to want to tramp through soggy fields; it's not Glastonbury.

As though to compound my feelings, Me and Bobby McGee just came on the radio and I was transported back to those nights in Ballymun when friends would call round with guitars and other instruments and we would play and sing and have a good time, and without any alcohol because we simply couldn't afford it. Ah halcyon days.

Followed by the Carpenters, Yesterday Once More.... Perhaps I should turn off the radio.

Perhaps I should try bingo. But we all know I'm not going to.

Monday 27th July 2009

I would like to report that this morning I have woken in a much better mood than yesterday, that my mood has lifted and I am no longer under a dark cloud of depression.

But that would be a load of shite.

Not only am I still feeling down, I am also bloody angry this morning owing to the fact that my neighbours were banging and crashing around until gone three o'clock this morning. I have no idea what they were doing, owing to my lack of x-ray vision, but it sounded as though they were rearranging the furniture.

Yesterday I tried to eat macaroni cheese again, but I didn't get half a can down before I started gagging when it hit the back of my throat, so today I am going to stick to soup. I have a small can of chicken soup ready. Cream of chicken, not chicken noodle as I discovered my chicken soup to be yesterday. When I emptied it into the pan I realised that I had bought the wrong soup and that this one was full of noodles and peppers. I don't think my throat is quite ready for peppers. So this is why I had to try the macaroni cheese instead.

Sometimes it feels as though I am never going to be able to eat again.

On top of everything else, I have now developed a rash on my face. It has the appearance of eczema and is very unsightly. I'm putting lashings of aquious cream on my face to keep it moisturised, and hopefully it will go away because it cannot be disguised with foundation. Make up only seems to exaggerate the dryness and with foundation it looks even worse. I have no idea if this rash is because of the treatment (the radiotherapy) or because of the drugs. But I can hardly stop taking the drugs just to find out.

Thursday 30th July 2009

Something happened to take my mind off my own problems on Tuesday. In the afternoon Tom was in the kitchen when he noticed Molly dog nudging and licking something in the back yard. It was a sparrow, a tiny baby sparrow who must have been trying to fly for the first time, but because there was something wrong with one of its wings, the poor thing dropped like a stone and landed just outside my kitchen door. It had twigs and string wrapped around one of its wings that had stopped the wing from developing properly. Once this was removed (Tom did it with scissors) it looked as though the wing was deformed, much in the way that women's feet were in China and Japan at one time.

It was obvious that this little guy was not going to be flying anywhere, but he appeared to be perfectly healthy other than the dodgy wing, so we decided to give him a fighting chance at life. I rang a few numbers, but in general people are not interested in the life of a little sparrow. Could it be that the smaller the creature, the less people care? Then I found Knoxwood, at Wigton, near Carlisle. They take in injured and sick birds from all over the north of England, so if the little guy were to have a chance, this would be the place for him to get it.

Overnight he slept in a small box in the kitchen window, and yesterday morning we travelled the 180 mile round trip to Knoxwood. We had already decided that if Knoxwood couldn't assure us that the little sparrow would be cared for and not killed then he was coming home again and would just have to live in a cage, like a little brown canary. But the girl who met us at the door took a look at him, examined the wing and told us that the wing *is* going to grow properly, and eventually he would be well enough to be released into the wild once more. She brought him into the building that is a purpose built hospital for little creatures and put him in with another sparrow.

And that's where we left him, chirping away, in the ward that contains little birds, a baby hedgehog, a couple of rats who were left out with the rubbish, a chipmunk and several ducks. Call me soft but I wish there were a way of telling his mum that he is fine now. The journey to Knoxwood wore me out, and when I got back I slept soundly for two hours.

Also on Tuesday, my wages were paid into my bank account in full. I should only have received half pay, not full pay, but it was nice to see my bank account looking so healthy for a while. I pride myself in my honesty, but even for someone as honest as I am it was tempting to say nothing. But if I did that I wouldn't be able to sleep with the guilt. After all, my employers have been very good to me these past few months.

Again on Tuesday afternoon (It was all happening on Tuesday) I had a phone call from a speech therapist, a woman called Lorna whom I have to see on the 7th of August. She is going to help me to learn how to swallow properly again, so that I can get proper solid food down. Ironically, Lorna is Scottish, and this is one accent I really have problems understanding; for me, my speech therapist is probably going to need to speak very slowly.

I don't have any pain in swallowing any more, and I am cutting down on the morphine because I need to function properly again. I have cut out the voltarol altogether, and I no longer need any medication to stop me from being sick. The mucus problem has almost gone completely now, and I no longer have to take tissue with me everywhere I go. My main problem now is the one that is going to stay with me even when I am completely healed; the dry mouth is something I am going to have to get used to, and am going to have to find ways of dealing with.

At the moment I have a glass of water with me at all times, and when I go out I either have a bottle of water or a spray container, like a little atomiser. The bottled water is more 'normal' as I find people look at me strangely when I spray into my mouth. The fake saliva has no better effect than water, much to my disappointment. If the fake saliva worked properly I would be able to eat foods that now stick to the inside of my mouth.

I have not used my tube for about a week now, so hopefully that will be removed when I visit the hospital next week. Although I am not eating properly yet, I am supplementing my food intake with Ensures. Much to my disappointment my taste buds don't seem to work on sweet foods at the moment. When I make Ready Brek I could put a whole pack of sugar in it and I still can't taste it; and it's the same when I have a black coffee, I may as well not bother putting sugar in. But that will improve with time. While my saliva glands may be destroyed for good, my taste buds will get better eventually.

In general, my condition has improved greatly, but mentally I still have a lot to come to terms with.

Friday 31st July 2009

I tried to eat shepherd's pie yesterday. The first bit I put into my mouth made me gag, and even though I persevered for ages, I didn't manage more than about 2 teaspoons of it, and had to give in before I brought what little I had swallowed back again. It was horribly depressing.

Nobody has told me whether or not this is how things should be at this stage. I have an appointment with Mr Small at Preston on the 4th of August, the date I am hoping to have my tube taken out, so I will ask then if my reaction to solid food is normal. Lorna, the woman who rang me the other day, was the one who suggested shepherd's pie with gravy, so I really did try.

It was such a disastrous attempt at eating that tears welled up in my eyes. Tears of frustration, disappointment and sadness all mingled together, but I managed to catch them before they cascaded down my cheeks. I so want to eat properly, but every time I try I gag. I don't want to live on Ensures for the rest of my life, so I hope that Lorna will be able to give me some exercises to do that will help me to get back eating again.

I should have seen a speech therapist weeks ago. I had a letter in the post to say that Preston had referred me to Barrow for this, but apparently politics have held things up as Barrow said I didn't come under their area, even though that is where anyone from Millom is sent when they need a hospital. But in this instance I come under west Cumbria, and so I have to go to Whitehaven to see Lorna.

I can't help wondering if this hold up has done some damage to my ability to swallow. Could it be that if I had this appointment a month ago, as I should have had it, I may have been given exercises to help that would have had me eating before now?

I took some ondansetron this morning. That's the stuff they give at the chemo department to stop patients from being sick, but apparently it also encourages the appetite. Yesterday, after trying to eat and gagging on the food so much, I felt really sick, so taking the medicine won't do me any harm, and if it encourages my appetite, so much the better. When I was going through my treatment there were times when I felt as though I could eat a three course meal, I longed for food so much. But now I don't even think about it any more. Yes I try to eat, but there is nothing I long for as I did during my radiotherapy. So I'm hoping that taking the ondansetron will do this for me.

Sunday 2nd August 2009

I can't stop crying this morning. I don't want to turn this book into a morbid tome about me feeling down, but that's just how it is at the moment. I don't know if other people feel like I do after having head and neck radiotherapy, but I feel so scared, so depressed, so bloody awful and I can't tell anyone how I feel. I don't want to upset my loved ones by telling them how bad I feel at the moment, but nor do I want to unload on a stranger who won't really care. I know there are caring professionals out there who are trained to deal with my kind of depression, but telling them how I feel won't make me feel any better. I am still going to feel bad because I can't eat anything above liquid, I am still going to feel terrified out of my wits that I may find further lumps, and if I do I don't think there's anything the docs can do about it. I am scared about so many different things on so many different levels, and I just don't know how to deal with it. Perhaps time will calm my fears that the cancer will return; only time will tell. Perhaps in time I will come to terms with the fact that I cannot eat the foods I used to eat; again only time will tell. The illusive 'they' say that you can get used to anything; I wish 'they' would show me how.

I went to the Macmillan website, to the forum, to see if there is anyone there who might be going through the same thing, but the forum is so sad that it just made me cry again. I didn't cry throughout the treatment, I stayed positive the whole time, yet now I feel like I am falling to pieces. I want to be told that the radiotherapy has definitely seen off the cancer, but as the doctors didn't know where it was in the first place, they cannot give me this reassurance.

I have started to reduce the amount of morphine I am taking; I have gone from taking 60mg of slow release morphine, morning and night, to taking 40mg. I have also reduced the oromorph from 3 teaspoons to 1. I wonder if this reduction could have anything to do with my depression. Again, I can't ask until Tuesday when I have my appointment with Mr Small.

I so wanted this book to be upbeat, to give anyone going through the same treatment an optimistic outlook, and here I am banging on about how bad I feel. Then again, these feelings are all psychological; the physical effects of the treatment are, as I have shown, manageable if somewhat difficult at the time. My psychological effects are mine alone, and I cannot say how anyone else is likely to feel mentally at the end of the treatment.

I don't think that being stuck at home is helping my mental outlook one little bit. I need to get back to work, to where I can converse with different people and feel as though I am making a difference in the world. But that in itself brings its own worries. Like, what am I going to take to work for my lunch. Something that was as simple as 'what can I put in a sandwich' has moved on to a whole new level. Whether or not I will be capable of eating sandwiches in the future remains to be seen, but at the moment there's not a cat in Hell's chance of me eating bread with fillings. The idea of soup for lunch every day is not something I relish, but then I tell myself that I should be grateful; there are people in this world who don't even have soup to eat.

Will I be able to cope with talking on the phone all day with a dry mouth? Obviously I will have a large glass of water on my desk at all times, but still it worries me.

Am I worrying about things unnecessarily? Is it because I am feeling down that all of these complications are piling into my mind? Feeling this down is alien to me, and I don't have any coping mechanisms to deal with it. I cope with feeling nervous by cracking jokes, but depression at this level is something that is new to me. Yes I have known intense sorrow in my life, but this is different, this is personal and I don't seem to be able to share it with anyone, so it is also a lonely feeling. At least I can write it here, where it's not going to upset any of my loved ones.

I really should give my head a shake and tell myself that I am so bloody lucky to be where I am right now. Health wise, I really don't feel ill, it's just the inability to eat solid foods, and I suppose that's not the worst thing in the world. I have a wonderful family, fine friends, a job to go back to with an employer who has shown care and consideration over what I have had to go through this year. Yes, I need to give my head a wobble and drag myself out of this quagmire of depression before it engulfs me.

Monday 3rd August 2009

Ditto as per yesterday.

Wednesday 5th August 2009

It is exactly a year ago today that my friend Alyson died, and this was the first thought on my mind when I woke up this morning. Around the time when I had my first neck dissection, Alyson went through a hysterectomy in South Africa. While

I was treated in the luxurious setting of Preston hospital under the National Health Service, Alyson was treated by a private hospital, and she had to find the money to pay for every procedure, every cotton bud used and she even had to take her own bedding into hospital with her. When the operation was done she was told that she would need some radiotherapy, but that she first had to lose some weight.

Alyson was a big lady, with a big heart, but I have seen people as big as she was being treated by radiotherapy at Preston. But in South Africa she was told that the radiotherapy tables would not take her weight. She tried to lose weight, but was unsuccessful, and so she decided to believe that they had got all of the cancer out with the hysterectomy. From time to time she would have a pain, like a stitch, in her side, but she shrugged it off and got on with her life, especially when her husband was head hunted by a company in Russia.

Although already in their fifties, they both took this adventure and ran with it, keeping their property in South Africa, just in case they should ever decide to move back.

But Russia was difficult for Alyson. Where they lived there was nobody who spoke English. Even at the hotel where they stayed before they found their own little flat, the only English voice Alyson heard was Roy's when he came home from work. Roy was supplied with an interpreter, which made life easier for him, but Alyson had to struggle, even to buy basic groceries. So when she became dreadfully constipated she had a hell of a job trying to get her needs across to a pharmacist.

Her pains gradually got worse, and Roy arranged for an interpreter to accompany her to a doctor at a hospital. To cut a long, drawn out story short, it eventually transpired that Alyson's cancer had spread through most of her lower body. It was in her bowel, and in her spine. The doctors could do nothing for her. It was too late for chemotherapy or radiotherapy, and all they could do was to send her home to die. She didn't know this, but I did because Roy wrote to tell me.

It broke my heart to know that Alyson was going to die without us ever getting a chance to meet in person. We had met on the internet, and this is where our friendship had been conducted over four years, along with little gifts in the post now and then. Two weeks before she left for a better place I rang her, hearing her voice for the first time as she told me that it would be at least a year before she would be allowed to fly again, to her beloved South Africa. It was heart wrenching to hear her words, knowing as I did that her time on this earth was very limited indeed.

Her pain during the latter part of her illness was horrific, and it was so hard for Roy to see her go through such pain. Because she was not a Russian citizen, Alyson could not be given morphine, as she would have been if she had been here. Her pain relief was not strong enough to cope with the dreadful pain that cancer brings in the latter stages, and so she died in agony. Even now this brings tears to my eyes, that such a fine lady had to go through agonies for want of morphine that is so readily available here.

Alyson's demise showed me just how great the chasms are between the care we are allowed in this country compared to that in many countries around the world. To anyone who complains about the NHS I would say 'be grateful'.

I had another monthly check up at Preston yesterday, and felt very grateful to be surrounded by so many caring professionals. There was a delay of over an hour before I got to see Mr Small, but that doesn't matter, it only serves to show that they give everyone the time they need, even if it causes a backlog of appointments. In Mr Small's office were also Dr Siva, Isabel the specialist nurse, a speech therapist and two nurses. Blimey, all for little old me.

The camera up my nose told Mr Small that all is healing as it should be, and that even though I am struggling to eat, he wouldn't expect me to be at any further stage at this time. I told him I have been feeling really depressed recently, and he said that this is to be expected too, that I have been through a huge trauma in my life and it would be strange if I didn't feel a little down at this stage.

I told Mr Small that coffee makes me cough, and he said that this is a good reaction to have, that coughing will help the healing process, and I think I can see what he means by this. Coughing must use up a lot of muscles, and so it must follow that it will help to make the muscles in my throat stronger.

Coughing doesn't help when I have a sore bottom from constipation, but I didn't think Mr Small needed this bit of information.

Almost in unison they all told me that I had done really well, and that I was continuing to do well, in spite of my feeling so low. Hearing this from the people who know their jobs so well went a long way towards lightening my mood.

After the consultation I went with Isabel to an office where she looked up her diary and gave me an appointment to have my tube removed next Wednesday. She is going to do it herself, and although she has warned me that it will hurt pretty badly for a moment, the pain subsides after about five minutes and it is a relatively easy experience. Still, I wish I could be sedated for it. I don't want to go through the pain of having it removed, but I so want it out of my stomach now.

I told Isabel how honoured I felt to have so many people taking an interest in my case, that it felt good to have to many people taking care of me, and how I didn't feel that I could have received such treatment if I had gone down the private health route. She pointed out that Mr Small sees so many patients that his expertise in the field is second to none, and suggested that perhaps a private doctor would not have the level of experience that Mr Small has. Again, a comforting thought.

Anyway, today I feel much more positive than I have been feeling of late. My cousin's wife wrote to tell me about a friend of theirs who had the same treatment about two years ago and is left with a dry mouth. They were at a dinner party with this friend the other night and while he ate slower than everyone else, he managed to eat the same food as the rest of the guests, so again this information gave me a positive outlook for the future.

But today is August the 5th. Today is Alyson day. Here's to you my friend, wherever you are.

Thursday 8th August 2009

Today is my parents' 61st wedding anniversary. Last week my Mum had a carcinoma removed from her head, yesterday my Dad had something removed from his ear, but as he won't tell us what the consultant said, I have no way of knowing what. Anyway, yesterday afternoon I went round to their house to see how he was after his little op.

There they were, watching Murder she Wrote as usual. Is there a channel specifically for Murder she Wrote? And I got to thinking… is that it? Is that what the poor working classes are destined for? Endless episodes of Murder she Wrote and the odd trip to the doctor/chemist/hospital? My parents are so old now that this really is all that their lives consist of. While I would happily take them out, this isn't what they want. Dad won't even go around the corner to the park for a picnic. He gets a taxi if he needs to go anywhere, which is really only on a Saturday when he goes to the post office to put on his lottery ticket and on a Sunday when he comes to visit me. Dad is so shaky on his legs, due to the fact that they are stick thin because he has no appetite, he can't make it to the loo without holding on to something all the way. Mum is scared to leave him for longer than it takes to slip out to the chemist to pick up a prescription, lest he fall over and do himself an injury.

It scares me to leave them alone, but this is what they want. Dad does not want anyone disturbing his marathon TV watching, nor does he want me there all the time because he can't smoke around me, and he smokes like the proverbial trooper he once was. My dad was one of the lost 14th army, in the Burmese jungle, fighting the Japanese for over 3 years. And yet to look at his frailness now, it is hard to equate the man he is now with the man he was then.

Anyway, the upshot was that I left my parents' house feeling all depressed again. I'm not saying that my parents' life depressed me in that they are unhappy, because they are not unhappy at all. They are quite content with their wide screen TV. Perhaps this is because they bothered to live their lives to the fullest when they were younger. They were always off out somewhere, be it only for a walk in the countryside. Mum used to love to bake, something that she doesn't do now because Dad worries that she might burn herself on the oven. Dad worries about all sorts of silly little things like that.

But what do I do with *my* life? Not much is the answer. When things are 'normal' I go to work, I come home and watch a bit of TV, I go to bed, I get up and go to work, come home and watch a bit of TV… Then at the weekends I try to catch up on a bit of correspondence on a Saturday, perhaps do a bit of housework, and on Sunday I try to entertain Mum and Dad for the afternoon as this is their day for visiting me when I am at work, and they like their routine. If it were not for entertaining Mum and Dad on a Sunday I could go off somewhere for the weekend in the motor home; but how do I let them down? I am their only child, and because I work so far away they only get to see me at the weekends.

I don't know why I wanted a motor home so badly. The furthest it has been since purchase is just up the coast to a little seaside village, and back again to be parked outside the house. In a couple of weeks time we are going away in it for the first time ever. Perhaps this is what I need to lighten my spirits because at the moment I can't get out of the doldrums at all.

Tom caught me crying last night, over nothing at all. Well, I say nothing at all, but it was because I felt so bad. My nose was blocked, which meant I couldn't keep my mouth closed, which meant that my mouth was drying up every couple of minutes. People on TV were eating, and it struck me how much we all take that simple action for granted. Eating is a natural thing, something we don't have to think about beyond what we like and dislike. But for me now eating is next to impossible, and even when people try to tell me that it will improve, that eventually I will learn how to cope with swallowing again, at the moment it's hard to believe.

I had no idea that this is what the consequence of a dry mouth would be. Yes Dr Siva had warned me that I would be left with a permanent dry mouth from the radiotherapy, but I didn't take this thought process any further, to the realisation that certain foods would be out of the question forever. Yes I was told that my throat would get so sore that it would be impossible to swallow, hence the tube in my tummy, but again I didn't think that this would be a long lasting problem. While I no longer have pain in my throat, my ability to swallow just is not there. And it's bloody depressing. The problem is compounded and set back when I try to eat, as in the omelette with ham, something simple, something that a normal person would have no problem with at all, and I feel as though I could choke. This takes away my confidence and I go back to the Ensures again, scared to try to eat for days.

Before I went to bed last night I only took 20 mg of morphine sulphate, the slow release morphine. Usually I can get off to sleep fairly quickly, but not last night. I lay there feeling as though my skin were crawling, until eventually I got out of bed and came back downstairs to take some oral morphine when I realised that this skin crawling feeling was a withdrawal symptom. Obviously I have cut down too far too quickly. I can cope with slight withdrawal symptoms such as this during the day, in fact the feeling would probably go unnoticed during the day, but I am going to have to cut down the oral morphine a lot slower that I have done. I don't need insomnia on top of everything else right now.

Tomorrow I go to see the speech therapist at Whitehaven. And I am hoping that she will be able to give me some ideas on how to cope with the eating, or not eating as is the case at the moment. I suppose, realistically, I could live on Ensures for the rest of my life without any ill effects. They give all the nutrition the body needs. Looking at the eating thing from another point of view, the consumption of foods is a 'want', rather than a 'need'. Need is covered by Ensures, want is looking at adverts for mars bars on TV and… well, wanting. There was a time, before the advent of mars bars, that nobody ate mars bars, and everyone coped just fine without them. And such is the case for most of the foods we are used to consuming. The advertising industry tells us that we need mars bars, and other such foods that once never existed, and we believe them because the taste of these foods appeals to our senses. But living without them, adjusting to foods that I *can* cope with, is not going to do me any lasting harm. What *is* doing me harm is feeling as though there is nothing to go on for; and excuse my colourful way of putting this, but that's just bollox.

I have so much to live for, and this isn't just me trying to pull myself up by the bootstraps. I have family who love me, grandchildren who make my heart swell with pride, and friends who care. It doesn't matter if I can't go out to restaurants, it doesn't matter if I can't eat particular foods, what matters is that I get better so that I can plan things to do with my loved ones. Life does not have to be an endless round of work and sleep. Yes I have to work to pay the bills, but that will not be forever. In a couple of years time all of the bills will be gone and I can start to save towards my retirement, which should happen in nine years time. Yes at the moment I am trapped in this gloomy little town because I can't leave my elderly parents, but eventually I will be in a position where I can sell the house and go off travelling in the motorhome, if that's what I want. Or perhaps I will be content to watch endless episodes of Murder she Wrote while I knit endless cardigans for my grandchildren.

Who knows what the future may bring? Nobody can be prepared for what is going to happen, but we can hope, and we can dream, and we can get on with living regardless of what obstacles are thrown in our path along the way. So my life has changed, albeit in a huge way that the majority of people will never have to deal with, but it is change nonetheless, and there have been many other huge changes I have had to come to terms with over the years, yet I have coped. Having to have all of my top teeth out to be replaced by dentures was one such change that I really could have done without. But I coped with it, and accepted that I would never eat toffee again. And I live without toffee quite easily. Now I have to live without a range of foods, but like toffee, I will just have to accept that I cannot eat potatoes, cheese, chocolate etc., and slowly find out what I *can* eat. Perhaps I will have a plain omelette while everyone else is eating their Christmas dinner, but then again, Christmas isn't about the consumption of food, it's about celebrating family, and I don't imagine there was a feast in the stable where Jesus was born.

Change happens, and while this change in my life is the most devastating so far, I will just have to learn to live with it, because there is no alternative other than feeling miserable, and who the heck wants to feel miserable all of the time? It's a horrible feeling, and the only way to get over it is to accept that things are different now.

Chapter four – a few years on

Still here.

I wasn't sure if I was ever going to come back to this, to edit it, and perhaps to publish it, but here I am having read through my own story, and ready to tell you what happened since.

Well, since 2009 I have given up trying to eat. I live on ensures; now and again having the occasional dunked biscuit; although, there's only one brand that actually tastes like a biscuit to me.

My taste buds have never recovered; I still have no sweet taste buds and most things taste really weird to me. I have never developed an ability to eat again, and at this stage I doubt I ever will.

The biggest change in my life is that my parents are no longer with me. Dad left this mortal coil in October 2010. His final days were spent dazed and confused in hospital, as he rapidly deteriorated. He was 87 years old.

For the next three years we would pick Mum up every evening from the bungalow she moved to after Dad died. Dad wasn't keen on spending money on what he considered to be buying for someone else, and so he discouraged Mum from buying new things. So when she got her bungalow I encouraged her to spend what Dad had left her on the dark red hall carpet she cherished, and on the new furniture to go with the new living room carpet that your feet sank into. Mum's little house was made complete by the arrival of Bobby, the cat that Dad wouldn't let her have.

Bobby was Minnie when he first arrived; only changing name at the same time as the information the she was a he was given to Mum by the vet.

And so life went on; Mum seemed to cope with the loss of Dad on the outside, but I reckon that inside she was empty without him, as much as we tried to fill up her time. We would go shopping together, and a few months after Dad died I took her to Dublin, for what something in my heart told me was going to be her last time.

Mum missed Dublin as much as I did, and it had been many years since she had been able to visit with her friends there. So that's what we did; we got on a plane and spent our days shopping and visiting Mum's friends. She had the best time; at least I think she did. Or she may have been wishing that I was my Dad.

In the evenings Mum have dinner in the hotel before we went to our room where she would catch up on the soaps while I put her hair in rollers for her. Sleeping in rollers is an art; I have no idea how she, or anyone else, manages to get a wink on sleep with them in. Mum could even sleep in the spikey ones.

It was a week I cherish in my mind. A week when it was just Mum and me. I rang home every night of course, but most of the time I was just spending quality time with my mother; I think it was as special for her as it was for me, I hope so anyway.

2013 was a nice summer that started early. We took Mum to a few country fair type of events at the weekends, where she would buy pots of homemade jam and marmalade.

Then on the 18th of June she went to bed and never woke up again.

She had been suffering from heartburn and from a pain in her left leg, so a couple of weeks previous I had taken her to the doctor. Her doctor didn't seem to pick up on the fact that the symptoms she was displaying corresponded with ischemic heart disease. A fact that I didn't know either until I consulted with Dr Google after

Mum died. I am still confused as to how Dr Google worked it out in seconds, but Mum's doctor missed the classic signs of heart trouble.

We gave Mum a great send-off, with all of her favourite music played at the crematorium. She had quite a good turn-out considering she wasn't the most sociable of women, she took a bit of getting to know, but once she accepted you as a friend, you knew you had found someone just a bit special. She didn't open her heart to everyone, her upbringing made her cautious, but when she accepted you into her life, you had a friend for as long as she was around. Even as her daughter I felt this friendship.

So, that's the biggest change. And it's all still a little bit raw, but I'm dealing with it, somehow.

Molly is gone too; a tumour caused problems that, in spite of surgery and every treatment available, she eventually had to be allowed to go. That morning, the day that we decided she had suffered enough, is ingrained in my memory as one of my saddest days.

What I am finding a little difficult to deal with is the 'illness', for want of a better word, that I have been left with because of the effects of the radiotherapy.

One side effect of the treatment I received is that I can no longer swallow properly, which means that occasionally I have developed pneumonia.

September 2013 I developed pneumonia again… or so I thought. I hadn't felt too well at work and so had left early. As I walked towards the station I noticed that my shoulder hurt when I walked, and when I breathed.

The only doctor available when I got home was a young girl, who I managed to convince quite easily that I had pneumonia. She gave me antibiotics and off I went home. But the pain when I tried to breathe got worse, so I consulted Dr Google, who suggested I might have pleurisy; and when I spoke to the doctor on the phone, she agreed and said to just keep taking the antibiotic.

I went back to work a couple of weeks later, but seemed to be stuck with a cough. Not coughing up anything nasty, just a clear mucus. I noticed that I puffed and panted if I climbed a flight of stairs, and when I got out of the shower, or got dressed, or walked to the back of the house to the bathroom (my house is tiny). While I have never been one for any form of fitness schedule, I was always fit enough for what I needed to do. I walked to work from the station, a walk of about a mile, so long as it wasn't raining, and back down again in the evening; it was the only exercise I got since Molly dog went to chase rabbits in the sky. But suddenly I found that I couldn't make it to walk up to work, up the slight incline of the high street. Walking back down was manageable, but I noticed that I couldn't say hello to anyone for quite some time once I got there, so completely out of breath that I couldn't speak.

I wouldn't have been able for the walk to the bus stop from the station, so it meant having to get taxis to work, then eventually I had to get them back down to the station in the evening too. The cough was still there, I was still coughing something up, I was breathless at the slightest activity, and assumed this to be some sort of after effect of the pleurisy. Dr Google said that it could take months to shake off the bitch of an illness that I consider to be far worse than pneumonia.

Anyway, to cut a long story short; my doctor diagnosed bronchiectasis. At first I thought he said bronchiecstasy, which I thought a rather contradictory term for how I felt at the time. He explained that my symptoms added up to a condition that can be the result of too many episodes of pneumonia. It seems the pleurisy was the straw that broke the camel's back, and I am now left with a permanent condition that I am going to have to learn how to live with.

But hey-ho! I learned how to live without toast!

On January 7th I came home from work feeling a bit ill. As the evening wore on I started to feel a bit worse and assumed I had picked up a virus of some sort; difficult to avoid when you work in an open plan office and travel by public transport. I stayed home on Wednesday and Thursday, and it was about 7 pm on the Thursday that I started to feel really ill. So I went to bed early, waking at 1 am with a temperature of 39c and an urge to throw up. When you don't have any saliva glands you don't get that watery mouth warning that you are going to be sick, so it becomes a little more pragmatic for me and those like me.

I felt truly dreadful, and quickly realised that pneumonia was imminent. I knew the difference between pneumonia and pleurisy, and up until that evening I think I would have preferred the latter; now I'm not so sure.

I couldn't keep the antibiotic nor the paracetamol down, so I couldn't get my temperature down. As the night wore on I got scared, and at 3 am an ambulance was called for. I was more than happy to head off to hospital, even if it was full of sick people, which was usually my argument for *not* going there when I got pneumonia.

Over the next three hours I managed to sip at paracetamol and got my temperature down by one degree. I decided that the ambulance wasn't coming, and I was way too ill to wait any longer; so I took myself off to bed, under the assumption that sleep is good for you when you are ill. Half an hour later the paramedics were walking all over my white bedroom carpet in their boots, after walking up the pale beige carpeted staircase in their boots. Well, you can't ask a paramedic to take their shoes off; it's just not right.

My temperature had gone down another half a degree, and as all my other vital signs were reading as healthy as a racehorse, they let me stay where I was.

I'm not a total martyr; I know when I'm ill, and I was ill, more ill than I can remember being since I was seven years old with pneumonia that they said should have carried me off. They said at the time that at least you can't get pneumonia twice. I have no idea where that piece of medical nonsense came from, but I do know that it *is* nonsense.

So I was off work the whole of the following week, and the week after that, and the week after that, until six weeks had passed in a blur of Jeremy Kyle, Come Dine With Me, The Waltons and The Little House on the Prairie.

Never have I been so weak and feeble.

During this time I have been to see a specialist about my bronchiectasis and have had a CT scan carried out. The specialist told me that he was going to put me on steroid inhalers. I told him that I had already tried these but that they made me so dry that I couldn't speak in anything other than a husky voice. My daughter said to look on the bright side; it would have been worse if my voice had become squeaky; and I suppose she had a point.

My doctor told me to ditch one of the inhalers; and my voice improved slightly. A week or so later I decided to stop using the other one because my voice was going again and I was developing thrush. It was so difficult to speak that I had to weigh up their advantages against losing my voice altogether.

I don't know how the specialist is going to take this news, but I did tell him that the side effect of causing a dry mouth is compounded by the fact that I no longer produce any saliva. My voice is slowly coming back, but I don't think I will ever sing again because of the breathing difficulties I have.

That may not mean much to people who don't sing, but to anyone who does, even if you sing rather badly, not to be able to do so is heartbreaking. I can still do it in my head, but I can't get the breath behind the notes to get them out.

The specialist told me that he was going to put me on steroid inhalers. I told him that I had already tried these but that they made me so dry that I couldn't speak in anything other than a husky voice. My daughter said to look on the bright side; it would have been worse if my voice had become squeaky; and I suppose she had a point.

My doctor told me to ditch one of the inhalers; and my voice improved slightly. A week or so later I decided to stop using the other one because my voice was going again and I was developing thrush. It was so difficult to speak that I had to weigh up their advantages against losing my voice altogether.

I don't know how the specialist is going to take this news, but I did tell him that the side effect of causing a dry mouth is compounded by the fact that I no longer produce any saliva.

I am also taking 6.5 ml of antibiotic every second day; the idea being that it helps to keep infection at bay. But with working where I do and travelling as I do, I think I would need a full body suit to stay away from germs and viruses.

I'm having another CT scan this week, this time with an injection of dye involved. Not looking forward to the needle at all.

'Just a little scratch,' they always say, though we all know fine well that it's a rare occasion when it doesn't feel like you're being stabbed with a Zulu spear.

Anyway, I'm going back to work on Monday. I have no idea whether I am able for it or not, and will not know the answer to this unless I try. I have to find out what my limitations are and do my best to work with them.

I'm getting a lift to the station from my house, I'll be getting a taxi to the door of the office where I work, and the only walking I have to do is from the train to the taxi at the other end, which I reckon is going to leave me quite breathless. There's a lift at the office, so that should make things a whole lot easier.

But still this work is not completed.

I still need to know what the results of the CT scans show. Because, of course, once you have cancer, every other ailment is a worry that it's back. No point in beating around the bush with that one. It's just how it is. If I get a pain in my big toe I think of Bob Marley. Anyone who has ever had cancer will tell you that even when they have been given the all clear it never goes away; once you have cancer the thought of it stays with you forever, kind of like a cancer in itself.

Also, it's not quite five years; it won't be five years until the doctor at the hospital says that they don't want to see me again. And then I shall panic, because although I am not mad keen on the camera going up my nose and down my throat, I do find in comforting that they are keeping an eye on what's going on down there.

Then I shall publish this work; although I'm not entirely sure that I should.

As I said at the start; my reason for writing this was because I couldn't find a book on the subject by anyone who hadn't died, so I had to write my own. Now I'm wondering if the whole story, with its not so happy ending, might frighten the bejaysus out of anyone who has to go through the same treatment.

When I say 'not so happy' I don't mean that I am not happy and grateful to be alive; of course I am. But the ending isn't perfect.

I will never eat again; when I was first put on the steroids I got hungry; hungry for something savoury; so I decided to try a couple of the sausages that you get in the tins of beans. And with a lot of nibbling and chewing I managed to get them down; two weeks later I was still coughing up bits of sausage.

Also, when I *try* to eat I am punished by horrendous heartburn.

It is living on a liquid diet that causes me to aspirate liquid that causes the pneumonia that eventually caused the bronchiectasis. Aspirating is what you might call a drink going down the wrong way. The body's reaction to this is to cough, but my throat doesn't work properly, so sometimes it stays down the wrong way.

A while ago I went on antidepressants for a while. It had to be liquid of course, and because my mouth is so incredibly sensitive, it burned like neat brandy, or worse.

I was still grieving the loss of my mother, the fact that I couldn't eat was really getting to me, and the cough was driving me nuts. I stayed on them a couple of weeks, and it worked, perhaps psychologically, like some kind of happy juice placebo, or maybe that shit really works. Because nothing has changed; I still miss Mum so much that I dream of her almost every night; I still want toast like I cannot tell you the longing is so huge; and I'm still coughing like crazy.

It's like an acceptance comes in eventually. Accepting that I will never see Mum sitting at my dining room table again is something I have yet to come to terms with. Even though I *can* see her there, if you know what I mean. But the not eating and the cough; I can either let them get me down or I can work at getting over it. I don't mean 'over it' as in developing an ability to eat or getting rid of the cough, because neither is going to happen. But I can accept that I am still here; and if you didn't know me, you wouldn't think, 'Ah, look at the poor sick woman.' You would still see a smartly dressed woman, wearing make-up and perfume, and always with nice shoes.

I don't look disabled, but I have to accept that I am. I can't walk 20 yards without having to stop to get my breath back and to cough in a kind of hacking way. If I sit still, I'm not so bad. If I lay on my left side, I'm grand, breathing away clear as a bell.

But I'm still going to go back to work on Monday. I need to be somewhere other than this house for a few hours a day. I spent most of this week baking cakes, not too physical an activity, but enough to show me that I can think, I can work, and I just have to cope with the getting there and back thing. A 50 mile round trip every day is no mean feat for someone with bronchiectasis.

I don't know when I am going to get back to this; perhaps when I get the results of the CT scan; which, I will admit, I am crapping myself about. That's one of the more difficult aspects of having had cancer; every test after that is a horrendous worry, and even when you're told you have something not very nice, like bronchiectasis, it's a relief it's not cancer.

21st April 2014

I wish I could report that I'm doing OK, but I'm not. I am constantly tired, I dread drinking my ensures because of how they make me cough, I have not been to work for weeks, and doubt that I will ever go back.

Depression is creeping back; each day is just a little harder to get through than the one before. It takes about an hour to get each ensure down, which means I am spending up to 6 hours a day just drinking ensures while I cough and choke.

Then there's the problem with my hands; whatever the hell that is.

In January, around the same time as I was suffering from the worst pneumonia I have ever had, I started to feel pain in my hands, particularly at night. Eye crossing, toe curling pain. I can still type, but there are so many things I cannot do, like open a bottle of water, or brush my hair. I can't grip anything without excruciating pain in my hands. My doctor has carried out blood tests, but there is nothing conclusive to say what this pain is.

So, yes I am depressed, and not sure where my life is heading at the moment.

I doubt I will be going back to work again; I can't cope with the travelling. I can't do anything without getting out of breath and coughing like crazy. Just going upstairs at night to go to bed is a nightly trauma I would rather not have to face.

I feel like an experiment; I don't feel like I received treatment in 2009, I feel that I was lied to, misled and misinformed. If anyone had said to me that I could end up with a debilitating illness, or that I would never eat again, perhaps I would have thought twice about having the radiotherapy on both sides of my neck. I don't know, because I wasn't told so much that it is impossible to guess what my decision would have been.

If I could eat, I could deal with everything else; I think I could anyway. Every social occasion, every day out, every holiday is all about food for the majority of people. I miss it, food that is. I miss food like I cannot even begin to put into words. Just to have a slice of toast, or better still, with baked beans on top, is what my dreams are made of.

Perhaps this is why I sleep so much; when I am asleep I can do all of those things that I can't do when I am awake. In my dreams I eat, I dash around, I breathe normally and I don't spend any time at all at varying hospital appointments.

I can sing in my dreams too; just like I once did in real life.

I know I should be grateful to be alive; and in so many ways I am. To watch my grandchildren grow and thrive is truly wonderful. To know that there is so much of life I cannot share with them is truly heartbreaking.

My granddaughter didn't have food at her 18th birthday party. I'm sure some of the guests thought it a bit odd that they were directed to the chippy next door rather than to the buffet. But I know why she made the decision not to have food at her party, it was because she didn't want me tormented by the sight of sausage rolls and pork pies.

29 April 2014

I am 58 years old now; it was my birthday on the 19th of April. I got 2 cards, and a bunch of flowers from a cousin. Birthdays are not like they were once you reach a certain age. Besides, how was I to celebrate? Cake? Champagne? A nice meal? Chocolates? None of those were appropriate, nor could I go shopping for the day unless it was online. Oh how I would have loved to go shopping then to lunch somewhere special. Instead, I ignored the day as best I could, the first birthday I have spent without my mother.

If I am sounding depressed… what can I say? Yes, I am depressed. I am terrified that I will have to live this way for the next 30 years, because I can't see anyone coming up with a solution to what makes me so depressed.

I really wanted to end this book on a high; I wanted to say how it is possible to come through throat cancer and to lead a full life afterwards.

That *is* what I am going to say. It *is* possible to be treated with radiotherapy as I was and to come through it able to eat. It *is* possible to go through the treatment and not to have the difficulties with swallowing that I have had. It *is* possible to come through throat cancer and lead a full life afterwards.

Not for me though. Not for me.

www.ingramcontent.com/pod-product-compliance
Lightning Source LLC
Chambersburg PA
CBHW060247290526
45789CB00001B/236

* 9 7 8 1 5 0 1 0 8 8 4 3 8 *